Quick Reference for
Pediatric
Emergency
Nursing

Colleen P. Andreoni, RN, MS, CEN, TNS
Trauma Education Coordinator
Loyola University Medical Center
Maywood, Illinois

Beverley Klinkhammer, RN, MS, MBA, CEN
Associate Vice President, Patient Care Services
Holy Cross Hospital
Chicago, Illinois

W.B. SAUNDERS COMPANY
A Harcourt Health Sciences Company
Philadelphia   London   Toronto   Montreal   Sydney   Tokyo

W.B. SAUNDERS COMPANY
A Harcourt Health Sciences Company

The Curtis Center
Independence Square West
Philadelphia, Pennsylvania 19106

Library of Congress Cataloging-in-Publication Data

Andreoni, Colleen P.
Quick reference for pediatric emergency nursing / Colleen
Andreoni, Beverley Klinkhammer.

p.   cm.

Includes index.

ISBN 0–7216–8327–4

1. Pediatric emergencies Handbooks, manuals, etc.
   2. Pediatric nursing Handbooks, manuals, etc.
   3. Emergency nursing Handbooks, manuals, etc.
   I. Klinkhammer, Beverley.   II. Title.   III. Title:
Pediatric emergency nursing.   [DNLM: 1. Emergency
Nursing—methods Handbooks.   2. Pediatric
Nursing—methods Handbooks.   3. Critical Care
Handbooks.   WY 49 A559q 2000]

RJ370.A53 2000   610.73′62—dc21

DNLM/DLC   99-35201

QUICK REFERENCE FOR
PEDIATRIC EMERGENCY
NURSING   ISBN 0–7216–8327–4

Printed in the United States of America.

Last digit is the print number: 9 8 7 6 5 4 3 2

Quick Reference for

Pediatric Emergency Nursing

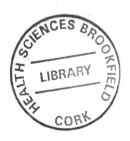

Reviewers

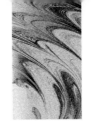

Megan Archer, RN, BSN, CEN, MICN, NREMT-P
Emergency Department
Carolinas Medical Center
Charlotte, North Carolina

Roselyn Holloway, RN, MSN
School of Nursing
Methodist Hospital
Lubbock, Texas

Susan Hopkins, RN, BSN, CEN
Ingalls Hospital
Harvey, Illinois

Barbara Weintraub, RN, BA, MPH, MSN, CEN, TNS
Children's Memorial Hospital
Chicago, Illinois

Jeanne Whalen, RN, BSN, CEN
Union Regional Medical Center
Monroe, North Carolina

Preface

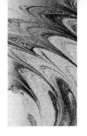

Emergency nurses must provide competent care to a variety of patients on a daily basis. Children are often our greatest challenge. Children comprise roughly one third of emergency department visits, except in tertiary care pediatric centers. The emergency nurse must stay current on the ever-changing aspects of emergency care for children as well as for adults. Textbooks on the specialty of pediatric emergency nursing are becoming widely available, but it is impossible to carry a large textbook in a pocket.

Quick Reference for Pediatric Emergency Nursing provides the reader with seven useful, concise sections that focus on the nursing care of children in an emergency department. The information will be helpful for the novice as well as the experienced emergency nurse.

This pocket reference provides quick information in a user-friendly format. It is a useful tool to serve as an adjunct to the knowledge obtained from basic and advanced professional education. It is not meant to be a primary source of detailed information. Rather, it is a primary resource for common to not-so-common pediatric emergency presentations, nursing procedures, medications, treatments, and pearls.

Caring for a child in the emergency department involves caring for the family as a whole. A critically ill or injured child not only requires our expertise in clinical skills and knowledge, but often a part of our heart as well. As emergency nurses we must never become so caught up in the technical aspects of care that we forget the **caring** component of our profession. Our children deserve to receive this from us.

"So, Mom . . . a good nurse doesn't need to know everything, just where to find it?" D. Andreoni, '98.

"That's right, son."

Colleen P. Andreoni
Beverley Klinkhammer

NOTICE

Contents

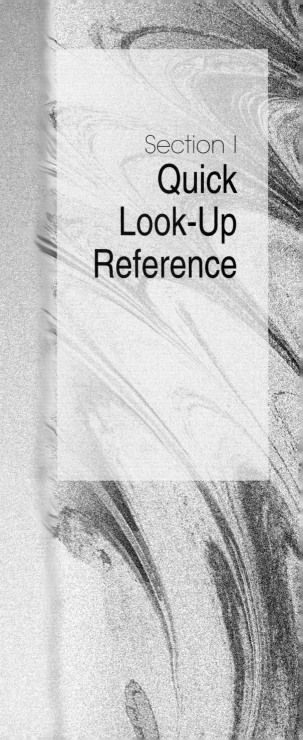

Section I
Quick Look-Up Reference

Reference 1. Determination of Apgar Score

Sign	0	1	2
Heart rate	Absent	<100 beats/min	>100 beats/min
Respiratory effect	Absent	Slow, irregular	Good, crying
Muscle tone	Limp	Some flexion	Active motion
Reflex irritability	No response	Grimace	Cough or sneeze
Color	Blue or pale	Pink body with blue extremities	All pink

From Tipsord-Klinkhammer B, Andreoni C: Quick Reference for Emergency Nursing. Philadelphia, W.B. Saunders, 1998.

Reference 2. Normal Values for Arterial Blood Gases in Children

Parameter	Neonate	1 mo–2 yr	>2 yr
pH	7.30–7.40	7.30–7.40	7.35–7.45
$PaCO_2$	30–35 mm Hg	30–35 mm Hg	35–45 mm Hg
HCO_3^-	20–22 mEq/L	20–22 mEq/L	22–24 mEq/L
PaO_2	60–90 mm Hg	80–100 mm Hg	80–100 mm Hg

Modified from Kendig EL, Chernick V: Disorders of the Respiratory Tract in Children, 4th ed. Philadelphia, W.B. Saunders, 1983, p. 148.

Reference 3. Asystole and Pulseless Arrest Decision Tree

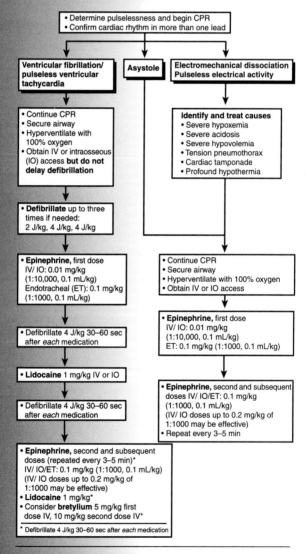

- Determine pulselessness and begin CPR
- Confirm cardiac rhythm in more than one lead

Ventricular fibrillation/ pulseless ventricular tachycardia

Asystole

Electromechanical dissociation Pulseless electrical activity

- Continue CPR
- Secure airway
- Hyperventilate with 100% oxygen
- Obtain IV or intraosseous (IO) access **but do not delay defibrillation**

Identify and treat causes
- Severe hypoxemia
- Severe acidosis
- Severe hypovolemia
- Tension pneumothorax
- Cardiac tamponade
- Profound hypothermia

- **Defibrillate** up to three times if needed: 2 J/kg, 4 J/kg, 4 J/kg

- **Epinephrine,** first dose IV/ IO: 0.01 mg/kg (1:10,000, 0.1 mL/kg) Endotracheal (ET): 0.1 mg/kg (1:1000, 0.1 mL/kg)

- Continue CPR
- Secure airway
- Hyperventilate with 100% oxygen
- Obtain IV or IO access

- Defibrillate 4 J/kg 30–60 sec after *each* medication

- **Epinephrine,** first dose IV/ IO: 0.01 mg/kg (1:10,000, 0.1 mL/kg) ET: 0.1 mg/kg (1:1000, 0.1 mL/kg)

- **Lidocaine** 1 mg/kg IV or IO

- Defibrillate 4 J/kg 30–60 sec after *each* medication

- **Epinephrine,** second and subsequent doses IV/ IO/ET: 0.1 mg/kg (1:1000, 0.1 mL/kg) (IV/ IO doses up to 0.2 mg/kg of 1:1000 may be effective)
- Repeat every 3–5 min

- **Epinephrine,** second and subsequent doses (repeated every 3–5 min)* IV/ IO/ET: 0.1 mg/kg (1:1000, 0.1 mL/kg) (IV/ IO doses up to 0.2 mg/kg of 1:1000 may be effective)
- **Lidocaine** 1 mg/kg*
- Consider **bretylium** 5 mg/kg first dose IV, 10 mg/kg second dose IV*

---
* Defibrillate 4 J/kg 30–60 sec after *each* medication

Reference 4. Using "AVPU" for a Brief Neurologic Assessment

AVPU

A = Child is *A*lert
V = Child responds to *V*erbal stimulus; i.e., calling his or her name
P = Child responds to a *P*ainful stimulus
U = Child remains *U*nresponsive to stimuli

Reference 5. Bradycardia Decision Tree

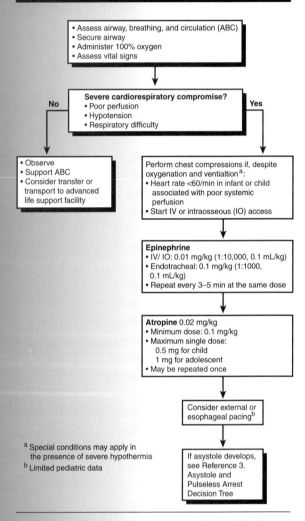

- Assess airway, breathing, and circulation (ABC)
- Secure airway
- Administer 100% oxygen
- Assess vital signs

Severe cardiorespiratory compromise?
- Poor perfusion
- Hypotension
- Respiratory difficulty

No

- Observe
- Support ABC
- Consider transfer or transport to advanced life support facility

Yes

Perform chest compressions if, despite oxygenation and ventialtion[a]:
- Heart rate <60/min in infant or child associated with poor systemic perfusion
- Start IV or intraosseous (IO) access

Epinephrine
- IV/ IO: 0.01 mg/kg (1:10,000, 0.1 mL/kg)
- Endotracheal: 0.1 mg/kg (1:1000, 0.1 mL/kg)
- Repeat every 3–5 min at the same dose

Atropine 0.02 mg/kg
- Minimum dose: 0.1 mg/kg
- Maximum single dose:
  0.5 mg for child
  1 mg for adolescent
- May be repeated once

Consider external or esophageal pacing[b]

[a] Special conditions may apply in the presence of severe hypothermia
[b] Limited pediatric data

If asystole develops, see Reference 3. Asystole and Pulseless Arrest Decision Tree

Reproduced with permission. Pediatric Advanced Life Support, 1997. Copyright American Heart Association.

Reference 6. Pediatric Cardiopulmonary Resuscitation—Basic Life Support (based on recommendations of the American Heart Association)

Action	Infant Considerations	Child Considerations
Determine unresponsiveness		
Activate Emergency Medical Service system/call for help	In absence of trauma, infant may be carried to phone while rescuer is initiating resuscitation	In absence of trauma, small child may be carried to phone while rescuer is initiating resuscitation
Airway		
Open airway by head tilt/chin lift or jaw thrust maneuver	Do not hyperextend infant's neck; neutral or sniffing position is preferred	
Use jaw thrust in presence of trauma		
Clear airway of blood, secretions, debris		
Breathing		
Look (rise and fall of chest), listen (air exchange), and feel (air escaping from child's mouth) for spontaneous respirations		

Continued on following page

Reference 6. Pediatric Cardiopulmonary Resuscitation—Basic Life Support (based on recommendations of the American Heart Association) *Continued*

Action	Infant Considerations	Child Considerations
If NO spontaneous respirations Deliver each rescue breath with only the force to initiate a visual rise in the chest Each breath is delivered over 1–1.5 sec Rescue breaths are continued until spontaneous respirations return or advanced life support measures are initiated	Deliver two initial breaths: mouth to nose and mouth using barrier device or appropriate-size mask with resuscitation bag	Deliver two initial breaths: mouth to mouth using barrier device or appropriate-size mask with resuscitation bag

Circulation

Assess for pulse

If NO pulse (or <60 beats/min with poor perfusion), begin rhythmic chest compressions

Chest compressions are continued until spontaneous pulse returns, until advanced life support measures are initiated by other personnel, or until lone rescuer is too exhausted to continue

Brachial
One finger breadth below nipple line
Compress with rescuer's 3rd and 4th fingers to depth of 0.5–1 inch
Deliver chest compressions at rate of at least 100/min
Five compressions to one rescue breath

Carotid
Heel of rescuer's one hand over lower half of sternum
Compress to depth of 1–1.5 inches
Deliver chest compressions at rate of 100/min
Five compressions to one rescue breath

9

Reference 7. Cerebrospinal Fluid Analysis Findings in Pathologic Conditions

	Appearance	Pressure	Cells	Protein	Glucose/Other
Normal lumbar CSF	Clear and colorless	70–200 mm H_2O	0–5/μL	15–45 mg/dL	50–75 mg/dL
Traumatic tap	Bloody; supernatant fluid clear	Normal	Red blood cells	4 mg/dL rise per 5000 red cells	NA
Acute purulent meningitis	Cloudy-milky or xanthochromatic	100–300 mm H_2O	Polymorphonuclear cells over 1000	Increased	Decreased early
Viral meningitis	Clear	Normal or increased	Zero to a few hundred, mostly leukocytes	50–200 mg/dL	Normal
Encephalitis	Clear and colorless	Normal or slightly elevated	Normal or increased	50–200 mg/dL	<40 mg/dL
Subdural hematoma	Yellow/clear and colorless	Increased	Normal	Normal or increased	Normal
Lead encephalopathy	Clear or slightly cloudy	Increased	Leukocytes	Normal or slightly increased	NA; lead in spinal fluid
Multiple sclerosis	Clear and colorless	Normal or low	Normal or increased	Normal or increased (increased gamma globulin)	NA; negative serology
Diabetic coma	Clear and colorless	Decreased	Normal	Normal or slightly increased	May be 200–300 mg/dL

From Ashwill J, Droske S: Nursing Care of Children: Principles and Practice. Philadelphia, W.B. Saunders, 1997, p. 1222.

Reference 8. Select Communicable Diseases

Disease	Incubation Period	Comments
Candidiasis	2–5 days	Communicable for duration of lesions
Cat scratch fever	3–14 days from inoculation to lesions	Transmitted through scratch, bite, lick, or other exposure to healthy cat; no direct transmission from person to person
Chickenpox	14–21 days	Duration, 5–20 days; contagious from 1 day before eruption until 6–7 days after lesions are crusted; rash begins as small, red macules; progresses to papules and then to vesicles
Chlamydia	5–10 days or more	Sexually transmitted
Conjunctivitis	24–72 hr	Transmitted by direct or indirect contact with discharge from infected eye
Diarrhea (see Gastroenteritis)		
Diphtheria	2–5 days	Characteristic lesion is patches of adherent grayish membrane with surrounding inflammation; usually in oropharynx; primarily found in unimmunized persons and communicable for average of 2 wk *Continued on following page*

11

Reference 8. Select Communicable Diseases *Continued*

Disease	Incubation Period	Comments
Erythema infectiosum (Fifth disease)	6–14 days	Macular rash, "slapped cheeks" appearance; lacy rash on arms and legs; may recur if exposed to strong sunlight
Food poisoning Staphylococci	30 min–7 hr	Frequently found in pastries, custards, salad dressings, sandwiches, sliced meats that have remained at room temperature for several hours
Botulism	12–36 hr	Characterized by central nervous system manifestations such as ptosis and visual difficulty, followed by descending symmetrical flaccid paralysis; vomiting and diarrhea may be present initially; frequently found in inadequately canned foods
Clostridium	6–24 hr	Sudden onset of colic followed by diarrhea; frequently found in food contaminated by soil or feces; associated with inadequately heated meats

Gastroenteritis (diarrhea due to the following)		
Escherichia coli	12–72 hr	Transmission through contaminated feces; perfuse watery diarrhea, abdominal cramping, vomiting; symptoms usually last <3–5 days
Campylobacter	1–10 days	Diarrhea, abdominal pain, fever, nausea, vomiting; usually self-limited within 1–4 days; organism found in food, unpasteurized milk; if not treated with antibiotics, organism is excreted for 2–7 wk
Rotaviral enteritis	48 hr	Seen in infants and young children; characterized by diarrhea and vomiting; transmitted by fecal-oral or fecal-respiratory route
Viral	24–48 hr	Self-limited, mild disease; nausea, vomiting, diarrhea, abdominal pain, myalgia, low-grade fever; unknown transmission—probably fecal-oral route

Continued on following page

Reference 8. Select Communicable Diseases *Continued*

Disease	Incubation Period	Comments
Giardiasis	5–25 days	Protozoan disease; diarrhea, steatorrhea, abdominal cramps, fatigue, weight loss; transmitted by ingestion of cysts in fecally contaminated water or food
Salmonella	6–72 hr	Transmitted by ingestion of infected food or feces-contaminated foods, including raw eggs, raw milk, meat, and poultry; also carried by pet turtles and chicks; symptoms include headache, abdominal pain, nausea, vomiting, and diarrhea
Gonococcal infection	2–7 days	Sexually transmitted; communicable for months if untreated
Herpes	2–12 days	Characterized by localized primary lesion, latency, and a tendency to localized recurrence; transmission by direct contact

Impetigo	NA	Bacterial (*Staphylococcus* or *Streptococcus*) infection; vesicular lesions; advances to yellow crust on a red base
Influenza	24–72 hr	Viral; transmission by direct contact with droplet; virus may persist for hours in dried mucus
Kawasaki syndrome	Unknown	Unknown cause; duration 6–8 wk; red maculopapular lesions; progresses to pruritic wheals; desquamation occurs within 2–7 days
Lice (pediculosis)	Eggs hatch in 7 days	Infestation of hairy parts of body; transmitted by direct contact with an infested person

Continued on following page

Reference 8. Select Communicable Diseases *Continued*

Disease	Incubation Period	Comments
Lyme disease	3–32 days after tick exposure	A tick-borne spirochetal disease with distinctive skin lesions. Lesions may be accompanied by malaise, fatigue, fever, headache, stiff neck, arthralgias, or lymphadenopathy; check recent possible tick exposure
Measles Rubeola, "hard measles, red measles"	10–20 days	Contagious from 4 days before to 5 days after rash appears; duration 10–15 days; rash is reddish macules; begins on face and spreads downward; within 1–2 days, rash is confluent
Rubella, "German measles"	14–21 days	Contagious from 7 days before to 5 days after rash appears; duration is 3–4 days; fever uncommon; rash is pink macular to red; begins on head and spreads downward

Meningitis		
Viral	Variable	Characterized by sudden onset of febrile illness with signs and symptoms of meningeal involvement; cerebrospinal fluid shows increased protein, normal sugar, no bacteria
Bacterial	2–10 days	70% of cases occur in children <5 yr; includes both meningococcal and haemophilus meningitis; transmission by direct contact, including droplets and discharges from nose and throat
Mononucleosis	4–6 wk	Infectious agent is Epstein-Barr virus; transmission is person to person by oropharyngeal route; fever, sore throat, lymphadenopathy are characteristic
Mumps	2–3 wk	Infective up to 7 days before and 9 days after parotitis; viral disease characterized by fever, swelling, and tenderness of one or more salivary glands

Continued on following page

Reference 8. Select Communicable Diseases *Continued*

Disease	Incubation Period	Comments
Pertussis (whooping cough)	7–10 days	Transmission by direct contact with respiratory discharges of infected persons; paroxysms characterized by repeated violent coughs followed by high-pitched inspiratory "whoop"
Rabies	2–8 wk	Transmitted by virus-laden saliva of a rabid animal; duration 2–6 days; death (if not treated) is due to respiratory paralysis
Rocky Mountain Spotted Fever	3–14 days	Transmitted by bite of an infected tick; characterized by sudden onset of fever, malaise, deep muscle pain, headache, chills, and conjunctival injection; rash appears on approximately the 3rd day
Scabies	2–6 wk	Direct skin-to-skin contact by mite infestation; the mite penetration is visible as papules or vesicles or as tiny, linear burrows containing mites and their eggs

Scarlet fever	1–7 days	Contagious during incubation period; bacterial group A streptococcus infection; fine, raised maculopapular rash; red strawberry tongue
Streptococcal disease	1–3 days	Frequent cause of sore throat from group A beta-hemolytic bacteria; direct or intimate contact with infected person
Tetanus (lockjaw)	3–21 days	Transmitted by tetanus spores introduced into the body by a puncture wound contaminated with soil or feces
Trichomoniasis	4–20 days	GU disease characterized by punctate lesions and a perfuse, thin, foamy yellowish discharge with foul odor; sexually transmitted; motile parasite infection
Tuberculosis	4–12 wk	Transmitted by exposure to the bacilli in airborne droplets from sputum of infected persons; communicable as long as the bacilli are being discharged in the sputum

Modified from Tipsord-Klinkhammer B, Andreoni C: Quick Reference for Emergency Nursing. Philadelphia, W.B. Saunders, 1998, pp. 26–37.

Reference 9. Pediatric Defibrillation and Cardioversion

Weight (kg)	Defibrillation (J)	Cardioversion (J)
4	8	2–4
6	12	3–6
8	16	4–8
10	20	5–10
15	30	8–15
20	40	10–20
30	60	15–30
40	80	20–40
50	100	25–50

Reference 10. Degree of Dehydration

Signs and Symptoms	Mild (<5% loss)	Moderate (10% loss)	Severe (15% loss)
Mucous membranes	Somewhat dry	Dry	Dry, cracked
Skin turgor	Normal	Decreased (poor)	Very poor
Anterior fontanel	Normal	Sunken	Sunken
Eyes (appearance of eyeballs)	Normal	Sunken	Sunken
Heart rate	Normal	Increased	Increased
Respiratory rate	Normal	Increased	Increased
Blood pressure	Normal	Minimally decreased	Decreased
Skin	Pale, warm	Very pale to cool, mottled	Mottled to cyanotic, cool
Capillary refill	Normal	Minimally delayed	Delayed

Modified from Barkin RM, Rosen P: Emergency Pediatrics: A Guide to Ambulatory Care, 4th ed. St. Louis, Mosby–Year Book, 1994, p. 60.

Reference 11. Volumes for Enema Administration

Age	Volume (mL)
Neonate	10–15 (use a 20-mL syringe)
Infant	50–250
Toddler	200–300
Preschool age	250–350
School age	500–750

Reference 12. Sizes for Selected Pediatric Equipment*

Device	Neonate (3–4 kg)	Infant (4–10 kg)	1–3 yr (10–15 kg)	3–9 yr (15–30 kg)	9–14 yr (30–50 kg)
Endotracheal tube (mm)	3.0–3.5	3.5–4.5	4–5	4.5–6.5	6.5–7.0
Gastric tube (F)	5	8	8–10	10–12	12–16
Urinary catheter (F)	5	8	8–10	10–12	12–16
Chest tube (F)	10–14	14–20	14–24	16–32	28–38
Suction catheter (F)	6	6–8	8	8–10	10–12
Blood pressure cuff	Newborn	Infant	Infant-child	Child	Child-adult

*Suggested sizes only. Consider individual child's size and clinical condition when selecting equipment.

23

Reference 13. Pediatric Modification of Glasgow Coma Scale (GCS) by Age of Patient*

Glasgow Coma Score

Eye opening

≥1 year

4 Spontaneously
3 To verbal command
2 To pain
1 No response

Best motor response

≥1 year

6 Obeys
5 Localizes pain
4 Flexion withdrawal
3 Flexion abnormal (decorticate posturing)
2 Extension (decerebrate posturing)
1 No response

Pediatric Modification

0–1 yr

4 Spontaneously
3 To shout
2 To pain
1 No response

0–1 yr

6 Normal spontaneous movements
5 Localizes pain
4 Flexion withdrawal
3 Flexion abnormal (decorticate posturing)
2 Extension (decerebrate posturing)
1 No response

Best verbal response

0–2 yr	2–5 yrs	≥5 years
5 Cries appropriately, smiles, coos	5 Appropriate words and phrases	5 Oriented and converses
4 Cries	4 Inappropriate words	4 Disoriented and converses
3 Inappropriate crying/screaming	3 Cries/screams	3 Inappropriate words
2 Grunts	2 Grunts	2 Incomprehensible sounds
1 No response	1 No response	1 No response

*Score is the sum of the individual scores from eye opening, best verbal response, and best motor response, using age-specific criteria. GCS of 13–15 indicates mild head injury, GCS of 9–12 indicates moderate head injury, and GCS <8 indicates severe head injury.

Modified from Barkin R, Rosen P: Emergency Pediatrics: A Guide to Ambulatory Care, 4th ed. St. Louis, Mosby–Year Book, 1994, p. 385.

Reference 14. Recommended Childhood Immunization Schedule

Vaccine	Birth	1 mo	2 mo	4 mo	6 mo	12 mo	15 mo	18 mo	4–6 yr	11–12 yr	14–16 yr
Hepatitis B	Hep B	Hep B	Hep B		Hep B					(Hep B)	
Diphtheria, tetanus, pertussis			DTaP	DTaP	DTaP		DTaP	DTaP		Td	Td
H. influenzae type b			Hib	Hib	Hib	Hib					
Polio			IPV	IPV		Polio			Polio		
Rotavirus			Rv	Rv	Rv						
Measles, mumps, rubella						MMR			MMR	(MMR)	
Varicella						Varicella	Varicella			(Var)	

DtaP, diphtheria and tetanus toxoids and acellular pertussis vaccine; Hep B, hepatitis B; Hib, *Haemophilus influenzae* type B; IPV, inactivated poliovirus vaccine; MMR, measles, mumps, and rubella vaccine; Rv, rotavirus vaccine; Td, tetanus and diphtheria; Var, varicella vaccine. Range is indicated by bars; vaccines to be given if missed are indicated by ovals.

Adapted from the Centers for Disease Control Recommended Immunization Schedule January–December 1999. Atlanta, CDC.

Reference 15. Pediatric Intramuscular Injection Sites

Site	Recommended Age	Pros and Cons
Vastus lateralis (anterior lateral thigh)	Infant to adult Preferred for children <3 yr	Largest muscle group in children <3 yr Can tolerate large injection volumes (0.5–2.0 mL) Area free of important nerves or blood vessels
Ventrogluteal (lateral hip)	Infant to adult Consider for children >3 yr	Can tolerate large injection volumes Area free of important nerves and blood vessels Easily accessible site
Dorsogluteal (upper outer buttock)	Contraindicated in children <3 yr or in children who have not been walking >1 yr	Large muscle mass in older children Can tolerate large injection volumes Danger of injury to sciatic nerve Exposure of site may cause embarrassment to child
Deltoid (upper arm)	Infant to adult	Small muscle mass Can tolerate only small injection volumes (0.5–1.0 mL) Easily accessible site Rapid absorption rate Danger of radial nerve injury in young children

Reprinted with permission from Emergency Nurses Association (ENA): Emergency Nursing Pediatric Course, Instructor Manual. Park Ridge, IL, Author, 1993.

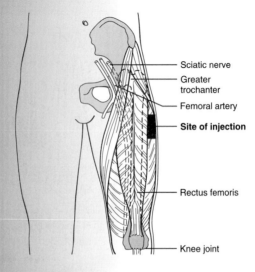

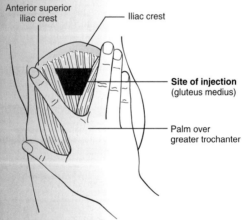

Figure R15–1. Intramuscular injection sites in children. (From Emergency Nurses Association (ENA): Emergency Nursing Pediatrics Course, Instructor Manual. Park Ridge, IL, Author, 1993.)

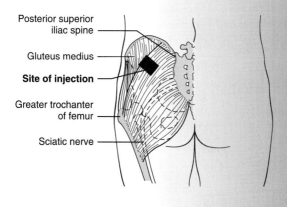

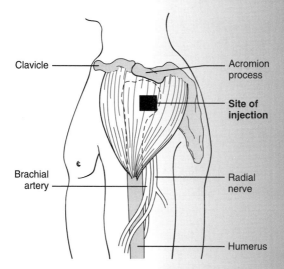

Figure R15–1 *Continued.*

Reference 16. Selected Normal Pediatric Laboratory Values

Test	Age	Value Range
Hematocrit	Newborn	42–68%
	3 mo	29–54%
	1 yr	29–41%
	3 yr	31–44%
	10 yr	34–45%
Hemoglobin	Newborn	
	1 day	15.5–24.5 g/dL
	4–8 days	14.3–22.3 g/dL
	2–8 wk	10.7–17.3 g/dL
	3–5 mo	9.9–15.5 g/dL
	6–11 mo	11.8 g/dL
	1–2 yr	9.0–14.6 g/dL
	3–9 yr	9.4–15.5 g/dL
	10 yr	10.7–15.5 g/dL
	11–15 yr	13.4 g/dL
Platelets	Newborn	100,000–300,000/μL
	3 mo	260,000/μL
	1–10 yr	250,000/μL
White blood cells	Newborn	9,000–30,000/μL
	3 mo	5,700–18,000/μL
	1 yr	6,000–17,500/μL
	3 yr	5,700–16,300/μL
	10 yr	4,500–13,500/μL
Glucose	Cord blood	45–96 mg/dL
	Preemie	20–60 mg/dL
	Newborn to 24 hr	40–60 mg/dL
	Newborn >24 hr	50–80 mg/dL
	Child	60–100 mg/dL
Sodium	Cord blood	116–166 mEq/L
	Infant	139–146 mEq/L
	Child	138–145 mEq/L
Potassium	Cord blood	5.6–12.0 mEq/L
	Newborn	3.7–5.0 mEq/L
	Infant	4.1–5.3 mEq/L
	Child	3.4–4.7 mEq/L

Reference 17A. Selected Medications and Drips

Critical Care

Drug	Dosage
Epinephrine	0.1–1.0 μg/kg/min IV
Atropine	0.02 mg/kg IV (maximum dose, 0.5 mg for child; 1 mg for adolescent)
Sodium bicarbonate	1–2 mEq/kg IV (maximum dose, 50 mEq)
Lidocaine	1 mg/kg IV (may repeat to maximum dose of 3 mg/kg)
Bretylium	5 mg/kg IV (may repeat to 10 mg/kg)
Isoproterenol	0.1–1.0 μg/kg/min IV
Magnesium sulfate	25–50 mg/kg IV over 20–30 min (maximum dose, 2 g)
Furosemide	0.5–1.0 mg/kg IV
Calcium chloride, 10%	20 mg/kg (0.2 mL/kg) given slowly IV
Adenosine	0.1 mg/kg rapid IV (maximum dose, 0.4 mg/kg or 12 mg)
Mannitol	0.25–0.5 g/kg IV
Lorazepam	0.05–0.1 mg/kg IV
Diazepam	0.1 mg/kg IV or 0.5 mg/kg rectally
Phenobarbital	20 mg/kg IV (give 1 mg/kg/min)
Phenytoin	20 mg/kg IV in normal saline (give 1 mg/kg/min)
Procainamide	3–6 mg/kg over 5 min (maximum dose, 100 mg/dose)

Drips (see also Section VII, Procedure 6. Calculating Inotropic Medications Using the "Rule of Sixes.")

Lidocaine	100 mg in 100 mL diluent
	1 mL/kg/hr = 17 μg/kg/min
	2 mL/kg/hr = 34 μg/kg/min
	3 mL/kg/hr = 51 μg/kg/min

Continued on following page

Reference 17A. Selected Medications and Drips *Continued*

Critical Care

Drug	Dosage
Esmolol	0.1–0.3 mg/kg min
Epinephrine	0.6 × weight in kilograms divided by 2 = mg drug + volume to total 50 mL = 1 mL/hr = 0.1 μg/kg/min
Dopamine and dobutamine	6 × weight in kilograms = mg drug + volume to total 100 mL = 1 mL/hr = 1 μg/kg/min

Reference 17B. Analgesia/Sedation Medications

Medication	Dosage
Fentanyl	1 μg/kg IV
Meperidine	1 mg/kg IV or IM
Midazolam	0.1 mg/kg IV or IM
Morphine sulfate	0.1 mg/kg IV or IM
Reversal Agents	
Flumazenil	0.01 mg/kg IV (>20 kg dosage is 0.2 mg)
Naloxone	0.1 mg/kg IV, IM, ET (>20 kg dosage is 2 mg)

ET = endotracheal tube.

Reference 17C. Frequently Used Antibiotics

Medication	Dosage
Ampicillin	100 mg/kg/dose IV
Ceftazidime (Fortaz)	50 mg/kg/dose IV
Cefotaxime (Claforan)	50 mg/kg/dose IV
Ceftriaxone (Rocephin)	50 mg/kg dose IV
Clindamycin (Cleocin)	50 mg/kg/dose IV
Gentamicin (Garamycin)	2.5 mg/kg/dose IV

Reference 18. Neonatal Resuscitation Steps Pyramid

- Assessment and resuscitation of neonate should occur simultaneously
- Procedures performed most frequently are at the top of the pyramid; most neonates require only the top-level procedures (i.e., drying and warming)
- Resuscitation progresses step by step (rapidly) down the pyramid

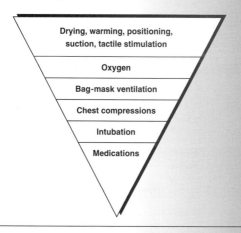

Drying, warming, positioning, suction, tactile stimulation

Oxygen

Bag-mask ventilation

Chest compressions

Intubation

Medications

Reference 19. Oxygen Administration Devices

Device	Oxygen Concentration (%)	Flow Rate (L/min)
Nasal cannula	24–30	1–2
	30–40	3–5
	42–44	6 (not recommended for younger children)
Simple mask	40–60	8–10
Partial rebreather mask	50–75	8–12
Nonrebreather mask	60–90	12–15
Venturi mask	24, 26, 28	4–6
	30, 35, 40	6–8
Tracheostomy collar	30–100	8–10
T-piece	30–100	8–10
Bag-valve-mask device with reservoir	60–100	15

From Tipsord-Klinkhammer B, Andreoni C: Quick Reference for Emergency Nursing. Philadelphia, W.B. Saunders, 1998, p. 217.

Reference 20. Wong-Baker Faces Pain Rating Scale

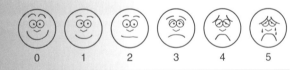

| 0 | 1 | 2 | 3 | 4 | 5 |

Face 0, no hurt; 1, hurts little bit; 2, hurts little more; 3, hurts even more; 4, hurts whole lot; 5, hurts worst. (From Wong DL, et al: Whaley and Wong's Nursing Care of Infants and Children, 6th ed. St. Louis, Mosby–Year Book, 1999, p. 1153. Reprinted by permission.)

Reference 21. Correlation Between SpO_2 and Pao_2*

Pao_2	SpO_2
100	97
90	97
80	96
70	94
60	91
50	85
40	74
30	57

*Based on the oxyhemoglobin dissociation curve, the SpO_2 may be correlated to the Pao_2 (assuming temperature = 37.0° C, $Paco_2$ = 40, pH = 7.40, 2,3-DPG level and hemoglobin level are normal).

From Tipsord-Klinkhammer B, Andreoni C: Quick Reference for Emergency Nursing. Philadelphia, W.B. Saunders, 1998, p. 221.

Reference 22. Pediatric Trauma Score*

Category Component	+2	+1	−1
Size	>20 kg	10–20 kg	<10 kg
Airway	Normal	Maintainable	Unmaintainable
Systolic BP†	>90 mm Hg	50–90 mm Hg	<50 mm Hg
CNS	Awake	Obtunded/LOC	Coma/decerebrate
Skeletal	None	Closed fracture	Open/multiple fractures
Cutaneous/wounds	None	Minor	Major/penetrating

*If score <8, refer to Pediatric Trauma Center.
†If proper size BP cuff is not available: +2 = palpable pulse at wrist; +1 = palpable pulse at groin; −1 = no palpable pulse.
BP, blood pressure; CNS, central nervous system; LOC, loss of consciousness.
Modified from Tepas J, Mollitt D, Talbert J, et al: The pediatric trauma score as a predictor of injury severity in the injured child. J Pediatr Surg 22:14, 1987.

Reference 23. Infant's Reflexes

Reflex	Description	Appearance	Disappearance
Babinski	Fanning of toes with upward extension when sole of foot is stroked	Birth	9 mo
Galant	Arching of trunk toward stimulated side when infant is stroked along spine	Birth	Neonatal period
Moro (startle)	Sudden outward extension of arms with midline return when infant is startled by loud noise or rapid change in position	Birth	4 mo
Palmar (grasp)	Grasping of object with fingers when palm is touched	Birth	4 mo
Parachute	Extension of arms and legs in protective manner when infant is held in a horizontal prone and moving-downward position	8 mo	Indefinite

Continued on following page

37

Reference 23. Infant's Reflexes Continued

Reflex	Description	Appearance	Disappearance
Placing	Attempting to raise and place foot on edge of surface when touched on top	Birth	12 mo
Plantar	Inward flexion of toes when balls of feet are stroked	Birth	12 mo
Righting	Attempting to maintain head in an upright position	Birth	24 mo
Rooting	Turning head toward stimulated side of cheek when touched	Birth	6 mo
Sucking	Initiation of sucking when object is placed in mouth	Birth	Indefinite
Swimming	Mimicking swimming movement when held horizontally in water	Birth	4 mo
Walking	Making stepping movements when held upright with feet touching a surface	First weeks; reappears at 4–5 mo	12 mo

From Betz CL, Sowden LA: Mosby's Pediatric Nursing Reference, 3rd ed. St. Louis, Mosby–Year Book, 1996, p. 542.

Reference 24. Salter-Harris Classification of Physeal Injury

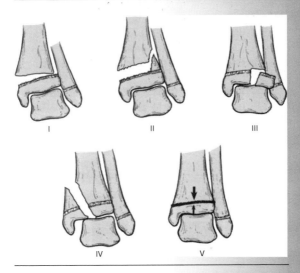

I, Pure separation through physis; II, metaphyseal spike; III, separation through physis and vertically through epiphysis; IV, fracture through metaphysis, through physis, and vertically through epiphysis; V, pure compression injury. (From Green N, Swiontkowski M: Skeletal Trauma in Children. Philadelphia, W.B. Saunders, 1998, p. 22.)

Reference 25. Classification of Hemorrhagic Shock in Pediatric Trauma Patients Based on Systemic Signs

System	Very Mild Hemorrhage (<15% Blood Volume Loss)	Mild Hemorrhage (15–25% Blood Volume Loss)	Moderate Hemorrhage (25% Blood Volume Loss)	Severe Hemorrhage (40% Blood Volume Loss)
Cardiovascular	HR normal or mildly increased Normal pulses Normal BP Normal pH	Tachycardia Peripheral pulses may be diminished Normal BP Normal pH	Significant tachycardia Thready peripheral pulses Hypotension Metabolic acidosis	Severe tachycardia Thready central pulses Significant hypotension Significant acidosis
Respiratory	Rate normal	Tachypnea	Moderate tachypnea	Severe tachypnea
Central nervous system	Slightly anxious	Irritable, confused Combative	Irritability or lethargy Diminished pain response	Lethargy Coma
Skin	Warm, pink Capillary refill brisk	Cool extremities, mottling Delayed capillary refill	Cool extremities, mottling or pallor Prolonged capillary refill	Cold extremities, pallor or cyanosis
Kidneys	Normal urine output	Oliguria, increased specific gravity	Oliguria, increased BUN	Anuria

BP, blood pressure; BUN, blood urea nitrogen; HR, heart rate.
From Soud TE, Rogers J: Manual of Pediatric Emergency Nursing, St. Louis, Mosby–Year Book, 1998, p. 503.

Reference 26. Temperature Conversion (Farenheit to Celsius)*

Farenheit	Celsius
96.8	36.0
97.7	36.5
98.6	37.0
99.5	37.5
100.4	38.0
101.3	38.5
102.2	39.0
103.1	39.5
104.0	40.0
104.9	40.5
105.8	41.1
107.6	42.0

*Formula: $°C = (°F - 32) \times 5/9$ or $(°F - 32) \times 0.55$

Reference 27. CIAMPEDS Triage History

Format	Questions
(C) Chief complaint	Why was the child brought to the emergency department? What is the primary problem or concern and duration of complaint?
(I) Immunizations	Are they up to date? When were they last given?
Isolation	Has the child recently been exposed to any communicable diseases?
(A) Allergies	Does the child have any known allergies? Is the child allergic to any medications? What was the child's reaction to the medication?
(M) Medications	Is the child taking any prescription or over-the-counter drugs (e.g., acetaminophen)? When was the last dose administered and how much was given? Is the child on immunosuppressive medications?
(P) Past medical history	Does the child have a history of any significant illness, injury, or hospitalization? Does the child have a known chronic illness?

Parent's impression of child's condition

What is different about the child's condition that concerns the caregiver?

(E) Events surrounding the illness or injury

How long has the child been ill? Was the onset rapid or slow? Has anyone else in the family been ill? If the emergency visit is for an injury, when did the injury occur, was it witnessed, and what happened?

(D) Diet

How much has the child been eating and drinking? When was the last time the child ate or drank?

Diapers

When was the child's last void? How much was it? When was the child's last bowel movement? What did it look like and how large was the stool?

(S) Symptoms associated with the illness or injury

What other symptoms are present? When did the symptoms begin? Has the condition gotten better or worse?

From Emergency Nurses Association (ENA): The Emergency Nursing Pediatrics Course. Park Ridge, IL, Author, 1993.

Reference 28. Normal Pediatric Vital Signs

Age	Weight (kg)	Heart Rate (avg/min)	Respiratory Rate (avg/min)	BP (sys) (mm Hg)
Premature	1	145	<40	42 ± 10
Newborn	2–3	125		60 ± 10
1 mo	4	120	24–35	80 ± 16
6 mo	7	130		89 ± 29
1 yr	10	125	20–30	96 ± 30
2–3 yr	12–14	115		99 ± 25
4–5 yr	16–18	100		99 ± 20
6–8 yr	20–26	100	12–25	105 ± 13
10–12 yr	32–42	75		112 ± 19
>14 yr	>50	70	12–18	120 ± 20

BP, blood pressure; sys, systolic.
Modified from Barkin R, Rosen P: Emergency Pediatrics: A Guide to Ambulatory Care, 4th ed. Mosby–Year Book, 1994.

Reference 29. Pounds to Kilograms Conversion Table

Pounds →	0	1	2	3	4	5	6	7	8	9
0	0.00	0.45	0.90	1.36	1.81	2.26	2.72	3.17	3.62	4.08
10	4.53	4.98	5.44	5.89	6.35	6.80	7.35	7.71	8.16	8.61
20	9.07	9.52	9.97	10.43	10.88	11.34	11.79	12.24	12.70	13.15
30	13.60	14.06	14.51	14.96	15.42	15.87	16.32	16.78	17.23	17.69
40	18.14	18.59	19.05	19.50	19.95	20.41	20.86	21.31	21.77	22.22
50	22.68	23.13	23.58	24.04	24.49	24.94	25.40	25.85	26.30	26.76
60	27.21	27.66	28.22	28.57	29.03	29.48	29.93	30.39	30.84	31.29
70	31.75	32.20	32.65	33.11	33.56	34.02	34.47	34.92	35.38	35.83
80	36.28	36.74	37.19	37.64	38.10	38.55	39.00	39.46	39.93	40.37
90	40.82	41.27	41.73	42.18	42.63	43.09	43.54	43.99	44.45	44.90

Continued on following page

Reference 29. Pounds to Kilograms Conversion Table Continued

Pounds →	0	1	2	3	4	5	6	7	8	9
100	45.36	45.81	46.26	46.72	47.17	47.62	48.08	48.53	48.98	49.44
110	49.89	50.34	50.80	51.25	51.71	52.16	52.61	53.07	53.52	53.97
120	54.43	54.88	55.33	55.79	56.24	56.70	57.15	57.60	58.06	58.51
130	58.96	59.42	59.87	60.32	60.78	61.23	61.68	62.14	62.59	63.05
140	63.50	63.95	64.41	64.86	65.31	65.77	66.22	66.67	67.13	67.58
150	68.04	68.49	68.94	69.40	69.85	70.30	70.76	71.21	71.66	72.12
160	72.57	73.02	73.48	73.93	74.39	74.84	75.29	75.75	76.20	76.65
170	77.11	77.56	78.01	78.47	78.92	79.38	79.83	80.28	80.74	81.19
180	81.64	82.10	82.55	83.00	83.46	83.91	84.36	84.82	85.27	85.73
190	86.18	86.68	87.09	87.54	87.99	88.45	88.90	89.35	89.81	90.26
200	90.72	91.17	91.62	92.08	92.53	92.98	93.44	93.89	94.34	94.80

Example: To determine the kilogram equivalent of 26 pounds, read 20 pounds on side scale, then 6 pounds on top scale. The kilogram equivalent is 11.79.

From Ashwill J, Droske S: Nursing Care of Children: Principles and Practice. Philadelphia, W.B. Saunders, 1997.

Reference 30. West Nomogram for Estimation of Surface Area

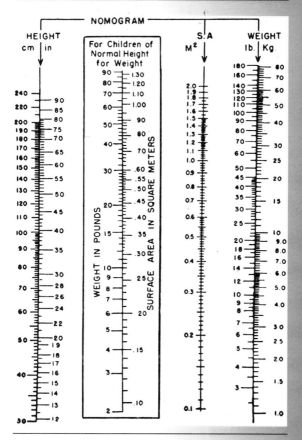

Surface area is indicated where a straight line that connects the height and weight levels intersects the surface area column, or the patient is roughly of average size, from the weight alone (enclosed area). (From Behrman R, Kliegman R: Nelson Essentials of Pediatrics, 3rd ed. Philadelphia, W.B. Saunders, 1998, p. 805; modified from data from Boyd E by West CD.)

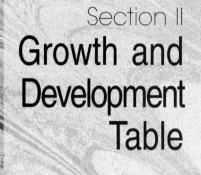

Section II

Growth and Development Table

Section II. Growth and Development Table

	Physical	Motor Skills	Psycho-social	Communication	Pain and Reflexes	Assessment Guidelines	Nutrition
Infant (birth–1 yr)	Period of most rapid growth Weight doubles by 6 mo, triples by 1 y Head circumference should be ~2 cm larger than chest circumference Anterior fontanel closes by 18–24 mo Posterior fontanel closes by 2–3 mo Distinguishes odors,	3 mo: can lift head in prone position 5 mo: turns from abdomen to back 7 mo: turns from back to abdomen; transfers objects from one hand to the other 9 mo: sits unsupported 12 mo: can walk with one hand; crawls quickly; sits from standing position	Trust vs mistrust After 6 mo, fears separation and strangers Coping skills: sucking, crying, cooing, babbling, thrashing	Cries in response to needs Most interactive during quiet alert stage Observe parents' interpretation of the infant's nonverbal communications By 1 yr, uses three-word vocabulary, one-word sentences Touch is important Responds to holding, rocking, patting	Does experience pain Withdraws from pain Reflexes: All present at birth Babinski—fans toes up and out when sole of foot is stroked; disappears at 9 mo Moro (startle)—sudden extension of arms and return to midline when startled by a	When possible, allow parent to hold child or maintain eye contact Allow infant to keep security object, pacifier Approach gently and quietly Use distraction techniques and objects Obtain rectal temperature and other intrusive examinations at end of assessment	No cow's milk during infancy: Formula or breast milk provide total nutrition until 3–4 mo First solid foods at 4–6 mo Rice cereal usually first solid Offer each new food over a period of several days before the next new food is given Generally, will eat every 2–4

Stage	Physical	Motor	Psychosocial	Cognitive/Language	Pain	Nursing interventions	Nutrition/Feeding
	recognizes mother's scent Visual acuity = 20/400 at birth; nears adult visual acuity by 8 mo Neonate bladder capacity: ~15 mL	12 mo: waves with wrist, uses pincer grasp, eats with fingers			loud noise or position change; disappears at 4 mo Rooting—turns head toward stimulated side when face stroked		hr until 6 mo Neonate: stomach holds ~90 mL Produces ~8 wet diapers per day
Toddler (1–3 yr)	Growth slows Average weight gain is ~5 pounds/yr Brain is 90% adult size by age 2 Anterior fontanel closes by 18–24 mo	Learning to walk 15 mo: able to walk alone, begins climbing Has a wide-based gait 24 mo: can dress self with simple clothing Can kick a ball without losing balance By age 2½ can build tower of six blocks and	Autonomy vs shame and doubt Expresses independence as "No!" Possessive of toys and parents Temper tantrums common Transitional objects may help separation anxiety	By age 2, can almost communicate verbally Attention span is ~2 min at 2 yr Believes what is heard literally Use short, concrete terms when describing or explaining	No formal concept of pain: may react as intensely to painless procedures as painful procedures Reacts with resistance, aggression, and regression Rare to fake pain Unreliable	Approach gradually, establish a relationship Allow the toddler to remain with parent as much as possible Let child play with equipment before using it on the child Use play to interact with	Decrease in appetite First and second molars and cuspids erupt Enjoys finger foods Using cup and spoon by 3 yr

Continued on following page

Section II. Growth and Development Table *Continued*

	Physical	Motor Skills	Psycho-social	Communication	Pain and Reflexes	Assessment Guidelines	Nutrition
		draw rough stick figures	Spends most of time playing Focus on potty training Very curious Fears: separation, loss of control, altered rituals, pain		answers when questioned about pain	the child Keep exposures minimal Praise the child for cooperation and when done with assessment	
Preschool (3–5 yr)	Gains less than 5 pounds/yr Growth in limbs more than in trunk	Dresses and undresses self Coordination and muscle strength increase rapidly Jumps rope, skips, plays catch	Initiative vs. guilt Greater independence Imitates parents and other adults Age of discovery Trial and error leads to learning	By age 6, beginning to understand cause and effect Over 2100-word vocabulary Using five-word complete sentences Counts to 10,	May think pain is a punishment Difficult to understand that painful procedures are necessary to get better All pain is perceived as	Allow child to be close to parent Allow child to handle equipment prior to your use Allow child to undress himself or	All 20 deciduous teeth are present by 3 yr; now starting to lose these teeth Learning to use a fork

	Physical	Motor	Psychosocial	Cognitive/Language	Reaction to Pain	Nursing Considerations	Dental/Other
		Learns to ride a bike Uses scissors, prints name, can tie shoe	Magical thinking May see injury or illness as a punishment Fears: mutilation, loss of control, death, dark, ghosts Coping skills: denial, somatization (usually GI), regression, displacement, projection, fantasy	knows days of week and name and address May benefit if given chance to ask questions Attention span ~10 min at 3 yr, ~30 min at 5 yr	"bad pain" Reacts to pain with aggression and, often, "I hate you"	herself, respect child's modesty Expose only as necessary for assessment Use play and games to elicit cooperation	
Schoolage (6–12 yr)	Gains ~5.5 pounds/yr Lymph tissue grows until age 9 Frontal sinuses develop at age 7 Beginning puberty in late	Musculoskeletal growth allows greater coordination and strength Involved in active play, sports, and games Performs	Industry vs inferiority Takes pride in accomplishments Interacts best with same-sex, same-age friends Becoming competitive in	Attention span >30 min Learns to write in cursive Beginning of logical thought Understands past, present, and future Growing	Reaction to pain often guided by past experiences Able to talk about pain in simple, descriptive terms May exaggerate	Help foster self-esteem by frequent and sincere praise Concept of health care is often guided by past experiences Allow privacy	All deciduous teeth are lost Will now have 26–28 permanent teeth Appetite increases Encourage dental hygiene

Continued on following page

	Physical	Motor Skills	Psycho-social	Communication	Pain and Reflexes	Assessment Guidelines	Nutrition
Schoolage (6–12 yr)	school age Increased myelinization provides improvement of fine motor skills	activities requiring balance and strength Beginning team sports Improved eye-hand coordination Learning new skills	games Remains dependent on parents for love and security Beginning to take responsibility Fears: separation from friends, loss of control, physical disability	vocabulary allows description of feelings and thoughts May be unable to verbalize need for parental support	pain due to fears of more pain or death	and time to compose self Explain purpose of the assessment, relating it to the child's illness/injury Diagrams and teaching aids are helpful Give older school-age child the choice of having parents remain during assessment	Ensure adequate hydration
Adolescent (12–21 yr)	Final growth spurt during	Greater coordination of	Identity vs role confusion	Memory fully developed	Accurately locates and	Give child the choice of	Dentition complete

childhood	gross and fine motor skills	Transition from child to adult	Able to project to future	describes pain	having parents remain during assessment	Orthodontia common
Experiences puberty		Peers are important and provide sense of belonging	Can see consequences of actions	May be hyperresponsive to pain	Explain the purpose of examination and all equipment	May alter meals/nutrition due to busy extracurricular schedule
Sweat gland function increases; acne common		Moody	Uses language to convey ideas, beliefs, values	Associates pain with possible changes in appearance or function	Allow child to undress in private	Often skips breakfast
Increased muscle mass		Developing own values	Language includes slang	Usually in good control during painful procedures	Provide feedback, especially normals, during assessment	Frequently eats fast food
Weight problems and eating disorders often seen in these children		Very private				
		Seeks independence				
		Family dissent common				
		Involved in risk-taking behaviors				
		Developing sexual orientation				
		Thinking of vocational goals, college				
		Fears: changes in physical appearance or functioning, dependency, loss of control				

Selected Bibliography

1. Betz CL, Sowden LA: Mosby's Pediatric Nursing Reference, 3rd ed. St. Louis, Mosby–Year Book, 1996.
2. Broyles BE: Clinical Companion for Ashwill and Droske Nursing Care of Children: Principles and Practice. Philadelphia, W.B. Saunders, 1997.
3. Engel J: Pocket Guide for Pediatric Assessment. St. Louis, C.V. Mosby, 1989.
4. Haley K, Baker P (eds): Instructor Manual Emergency Nursing Pediatric Course. Chicago, Emergency Nurses Association, 1993.

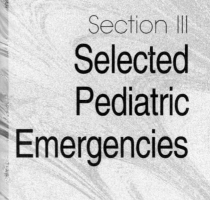

Section III
Selected Pediatric Emergencies

Chapter 1
Cardiovascular

CONGENITAL HEART DISEASES

- Major cause of death within the 1st year of life
- More likely to have extracardiac defects (e.g., tracheoesophageal fistula, renal agenesis, diaphragmatic hernias)

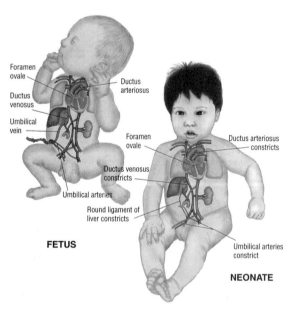

Figure 1–1. Changes in circulation at birth. (From Ashwill J, Droske S: Nursing Care of Children: Principles and Practice. Philadelphia, W.B. Saunders, 1997, p. 910.)

Acyanotic Defects

- Usually involves left-to-right shunting through an abnormal opening
  - Examples of left-to-right shunts include
    - Patent ductus arteriosus (PDA)
      - May have widened pulse pressure and bounding pulses
      - Administration of prostaglandin inhibitor may be successful in newborns
    - Atrial septal defect (ASD)
      - May be at risk for atrial dysrhythmias
      - Surgical closure necessary for moderate to large defects
    - Ventricular septal defect (VSD)
      - May vary in size from very small hole to absence of the septum
      - Palliative treatment includes pulmonary banding in infants
    - Complete atrioventricular canal defect (CAVCD)
      - Infants are usually small, appear undernourished, often have frequent upper respiratory infections
      - Palliative treatment includes pulmonary artery banding in infants
- May be caused by obstructive lesion that produces a reduction of blood flow to body
  - Examples of obstructive lesions include
    - Aortic stenosis (AS)
      - Faint pulses, hypotension, tachycardia, poor feeding
    - Pulmonic stenosis (PS)
      - Poor exercise tolerance, episodes of chest pain, dizziness with prolonged standing
    - Coarctation of the aorta (COA)
      - High blood pressure in arms, weak or absent femoral pulses, lower blood pressure in lower extremities
      - Infants may present with congestive heart failure (CHF)

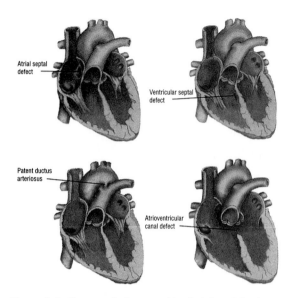

Figure 1–2. Common lesions resulting in left-to-right shunts. (From Ashwill J, Droske S: Nursing Care of Children: Principles and Practice. Philadelphia, W.B. Saunders, 1997, p. 916.)

- Older child may present with dizziness, headache, syncope
- All acyanotic defects have a characteristic murmur

Cyanotic Defects

- Usually involves right-to-left shunting through an abnormal opening
- Examples include
  - Tetralogy of Fallot (TOF)
    - Includes four defects
      - VSD
      - PS
      - Overriding aorta
      - Right ventricular hypertrophy

- Characterized by acute episodes of cyanosis and hypoxia (blue spells or "tet" spells)
      - Palliative treatment includes Blalock-Taussig procedure
- Transposition of great vessels (TGV)
  - May have no audible murmur
  - Between 2 and 4 wk of age, commonly presents with signs and symptoms of CHF
- Truncus arteriosus (TA)
  - Signs and symptoms of CHF
  - Visible cyanosis
  - Poor growth and exercise intolerance

CONGESTIVE HEART FAILURE

- Congenital heart disease is the most common cause of CHF in infants
- Diseases that impair myocardial function are the most common causes after age 1 yr
  - Rheumatic heart disease
  - Endocarditis
  - Cardiomyopathy
  - Dysrhythmias
- In infants, important early finding is often poor feedings
  - Taking a long time to feed, tachypneic and/or diaphoretic during feeding
- Signs and symptoms
  - Tachypnea (>60), retractions, nasal flaring
  - Hepatomegaly
  - Edema, usually periorbital in infants
  - Jugular vein distention (JVD) often not visible because of short, fat neck of infant
  - Chest x-ray reveals cardiomegaly
  - Oxygen therapy used with caution in left-to-right shunts, as it may increase pulmonary blood flow
    - Do administer oxygen with saturation <80% and with pulmonary edema
- Pharmacologic agents used
  - Digoxin

- Furosemide
- Bumetanide
- Metolazone
- Spironolactone
- Sodium nitroprusside
- Captopril

KAWASAKI DISEASE

- Produces multisystem vasculitis
- Infants <1 yr of age at greatest risk for cardiac involvement
- Death usually caused by coronary thrombosis or severe scar formation and stenosis of the main coronary artery
- Peak incidence between 18 and 24 mo of age
- Three phases
  - Acute (lasts 8–15 days)
    - Characterized by
      - Abrupt-onset high fever unresponsive to antibiotics and antipyretics
      - Irritability
      - Edema and redness of hands and feet
      - Rashes
      - Conjunctival irritation
      - Strawberry tongue
      - Cracked, red lips
      - Diffuse erythema of oral pharynx
  - Subacute (lasts 10–25 days)
    - Resolution of fever and other findings
    - Desquamation of fingers and toes
    - Time of greatest risk for development for coronary artery aneurysms
  - Convalescent phase
    - All clinical signs have resolved
- Will require 6–8 weeks from onset of symptoms for laboratory values to return to normal
  - Erythrocyte sedimentation rate
  - C-reactive protein
  - Platelet count
  - Urinalysis

- Treatment includes
  - High-dose IV gamma globulin
    - Single large infusion 2 g/kg over 8–10 hr
  - Aspirin
    - Initially in anti-inflammatory doses of 80–100 mg/kg/day in divided doses q 6 hr
    - In subacute phase, aspirin given as anti-platelet dose of 3–5 mg/kg/day

SUPRAVENTRICULAR TACHYCARDIA (SVT)

- Ventricular filling time is decreased, resulting in decreased cardiac output
- Narrow complex tachycardia, 90% of pediatric dysrhythmias
- Heart rates can vary between 200 and 300 beats/min
- Onset may be sudden
- Symptoms may be mild to severe

Emergency Department Treatment for Stable Child with SVT

- Vagal maneuvers
- Adenosine rapid IV push at most proximal injection port
  - 0.1 mg/kg/dose, immediately followed with 2–3 mL normal saline
  - If no effect, may double the dose and repeat once; maximum dose, 12 mg (see Reference 17A. Selected Medications and Drips)
- Digoxin
- Verapamil, 0.1 mg/kg/bolus; may be given to children >1 yr of age

Emergency Department Treatment for Unstable Child with SVT

- Immediate synchronized cardioversion 0.5–1 J/kg

- May double subsequent doses up to 10 J/kg
- Cardioversion not recommended if child has received digoxin
  - Ventricular dysrhythmias or sinoatrial node failure may occur
- Esophageal or right atrial overdrive pacing may be indicated

Selected Bibliography

American Heart Association: Textbook of Pediatric Advanced Life Support. Dallas, Scientific Publishing, 1994.

Ashwill J, Droske S: Nursing Care of Children: Principles and Practice. Philadelphia, W.B. Saunders, 1997.

Betz C, Sowden L: Mosby's Pediatric Nursing Reference, 3rd ed. St. Louis, Mosby–Year Book, 1996.

Chapter 2
Endocrine

DIABETES MELLITUS (DM)

- Type 1 insulin-dependent DM (IDDM)
  - Juvenile-onset DM is generally IDDM
    - Mean onset between ages 10 and 13 yr
  - IDDM can occur at any age
- Type 2 non–insulin-dependent DM (NIDDM)
  - Onset is generally after age 40 yr
- Islands of Langerhans in pancreas have major functions
  - Alpha cells produce glucagon by stimulating the liver to release stored glucose (glycogenolysis)
  - Beta cells produce insulin, which helps glucose enter the cells for metabolism
  - Delta cells produce somatostatin, which helps regulate insulin and glucagon release into the cells
- In DM, there is a dysfunction in the pancreatic hormone production
- Counterregulatory hormones mobilize and increase glucose levels
  - Growth hormones
  - Glucagon
  - Epinephrine
  - Cortisol

Signs and Symptoms

- Excessive thirst
- Polyuria
- Weakness and fatigue
- Weight loss, even with increased food consumption
  - Infants may exhibit feeding difficulty

- Decreased resistance to infections
- Dry, pruritic skin
- Blurred vision
- Abdominal pain
- Fruity breath
- Signs of dehydration
- Irritability or fussiness
- Lethargy
- Girls may exhibit vaginal yeast infection
- Many long-term effects
  - Growth delay
  - Recurrent infections
  - Neuropathy
  - Systemic effects due to protein entrapment on the walls of blood vessels by glycosyl radicals
    - Renal
    - Heart
    - Eye

DIABETIC KETOACIDOSIS (DKA)

- Produces osmotic diuresis
- Results in systemic dehydration
- Lipolysis and protein catabolism produce cellular energy
  - Ketones are the byproduct
- Hyperventilation occurs to compensate for metabolic acidosis

HYPERGLYCEMIC HYPEROSMOLAR NONKETOTIC COMA

- More common in older persons with NIDDM who may or may not already be diagnosed
- Generally indicative of a chronic problem that is precipitated by an acute infection or sepsis
- Dehydration due to hyperglycemia
- Osmotic diuresis occurs, as in DKA
- No ketoacidosis, because of the presence of enough endogenous insulin

- Serum glucose levels are usually very high (often >1000 mg/dL)
- Generally takes much less insulin to correct the problem

HYPOGLYCEMIA

- Caused by an oversupply of insulin or increased usage of glucose
  - Results in decreased glucose availability
- Infants and children have the greatest need for glucose
  - Higher basal metabolic rate
  - Required for growth
  - Larger brain-to-body size than adults
    - Central nervous system requires constant supply of glucose
- Somogyi effect
  - Occurs when glucose levels fall to the point where the counterregulatory hormones are released
  - Causes *rebound* hyperglycemia
    - Treated by increasing food intake and/or decreasing insulin

EMERGENCY DEPARTMENT TREATMENT

- Airway, breathing, and circulation
- Establish IV access
  - Rehydration
- Complete blood count, chemistry, glycosylated hemoglobin, urinalysis, serum acetone
  - Point-of-care testing can include fingerstick glucose, urine dipstick (look for ketones)
- Arterial blood gas to determine acid-base status
- Treatment for hypoglycemia, hyperglycemia, DKA, as indicated (see Tables 2–1 to 2–3)

Table 2–1. Insulin Drip Protocol for DKA

How/What	Why
• Mix 100 mL 0.9% NaCl with 10 units regular insulin	• Produces a solution concentration of 1 mL = 0.1 unit
• Weigh child in kilograms	• Weight in kilograms needed to figure accurate insulin drip formula based on the above concentration
• Purge the IV tubing set with a minimum of 20 mL insulin solution	• Insulin is absorbed by glass and polyvinylchloride, and as much as 60% of insulin can be lost to equipment
• Use an infusion pump for insulin drip delivery	• Prevents runaway infusion
• Set pump to desired rate	• 1 mL (0.1 unit) × weight of child in kilograms = mL/hr *Example:* 25-kg child 1 mL (0.1 unit) × 25 kg = 25 mL/hr/pump
• Monitor the rate of glucose fall to stay within 50–100 mg/dL/hr	• Fluid shifts can lead to cerebral edema
• Add dextrose, 5%, to IV solution when blood glucose reaches 250 mg/dL	• Prevents hypoglycemia and speeds up the resolution of ketone bodies by decreasing lipolysis
• If glucose drops below 150 mg/dL, decrease the insulin drip to 0.05 unit/kg/hr and then titrate to keep glucose between 100 and 200 mg/dL	• Same as above
• Administer subcutaneous regular- and intermediate-acting insulins 30–40 min before discontinuing the insulin drip	• The half-life of insulin is short; the subcutaneous injection helps prevent rebound hyperglycemia and acidosis

Table 2-2. Insulin Types

Name	Onset	Peak	Duration
Regular (Humulin-R, Novolin-R, Iletin I, Iletin II, Regular Iletin I, II, Regular Purified Pork Insulin, Velosulin)	0.5–1.0 hr	2–5 hr	5–8 hr
Prompt insulin zinc suspension (Semilente Insulin, Semilente Iletin I, Semilente Purified Pork)	1–2 hr	5–10 hr	12–16 hr
Isophane insulin suspension (NPH, Humulin-N), Insulatard NPH, Insulatard NPH Human, Iletin NPH, Iletin II NPH, Novalin-N, NPH-N)	1–2 hr	4–12 hr	24–48 hr
Protamine zinc insulin suspension (Protamine Zinc Iletin I, II)	4–8 hr	14–24 hr	36 hr or more
Extended insulin zinc suspension (Ultralente, Humulin-U)	4–8 hr	10–30 hr	36 hr or more
Isophane insulin suspension and regular insulin (Humulin 70/30, Novolin 70/30)	0.25–1.0 hr	2–8 hr	24 hr
Insulin analog (Humalog)	15 min	40–60 min	Variable Half-life is 46 min

Adapted from Tipsord-Klinkhammer B, Andreoni C: Quick Reference for Emergency Nursing. Philadelphia, W.B. Saunders, 1998.

Table 2–3. Treatment of Hypoglycemia

Age	Drug	Intravenous/Intraosseous Solution
Neonate	Dextrose 10%, 3–5 mL/kg bolus slowly over 2 min	Dextrose 10% in water; maintenance rate by infusion pump
Child	Dextrose 25%, 1–2 mL/kg rapid IV bolus	Dextrose 5% in water; maintenance rate by infusion pump
Neonate and child	Glucagon 0.1 mg/kg Maximum dose, 1 mg	Given when IV or IO access is unavailable

Mild hypoglycemia
Can be treated with foods (crackers, bread, peanut butter, or candy); juices or milk; or dextrose 5% oral solution (for infants)
The symptoms must be mild without signs of mental status changes
The child must be able to cooperate by eating and drinking
Never try to treat hypoglycemia with food or drink in an unresponsive child

Selected Bibliography

Betz C, Sowden L: Mosby's Pediatric Nursing Reference, 3rd ed. St. Louis, Mosby–Year Book, 1996.

Behrman R, Kliegman R: Nelson Essentials of Pediatrics, 3rd ed. Philadelphia, W.B. Saunders, 1998.

Soud T, Rogers J: Manual of Pediatric Emergency Nursing. St. Louis, Mosby-Year Book, 1998.

Tipsord-Klinkhammer B, Andreoni C: Quick Reference for Emergency Nursing. Philadelphia, W.B. Saunders, 1998.

Chapter 3
Environmental Emergencies

THERMAL EMERGENCIES

Burns

- Morbidity and mortality relate to child's age
  - Very young children have higher risk
    - Skin is thinner
    - Larger body surface area
      - Higher risk for fluid loss, heat loss, dehydration

SOURCE OF BURN

- Thermal
  - Most common in children
    - A leading cause of accidental death
  - <5 yr old: scald burns
  - >5 yr old: flame burns
  - Causes:
    - Flame
    - Hot liquid
- Electrical
  - Extent of injury determined by
    - Source of current (AC or DC)
    - Voltage
    - Path of current through body
    - Occurrence of arc
    - Type of grounding
    - High-risk electrical burn lesion
      - Left arm: May indicate myocardial damage
      - Head: May indicate damage to brain, spinal cord, or ocular lens
- Chemical

- Causes
  - Strong alkalis or acids
  - Alkali burns are more serious
- Extent of injury determined by
  - Mechanism of action of chemical
  - Duration of contact
  - Inhalation
  - Surface area exposed
- Special considerations
  - Do not initially look for antidote; immediately flush with copious amounts of water
  - Remove all clothing in contact with chemical
  - Brush away solid chemical
- Lime
  - Brush away dry lime before washing lesions
- Strong acids
  - If pain persists after initial flushing, apply a solution of sodium bicarbonate, magnesium hydroxide, or common soap
- Strong alkalis
  - Continuously flush area for prolonged period

ZONES OF INJURY

- Zone of necrosis/coagulopathy
  - Tissue irreversibly destroyed by injury
- Zone of stasis/ischemia
  - Adjacent to zone of necrosis
  - Tissue damaged
  - May recover or become necrotic
- Zone of hyperemia/inflammation
  - Tissue not injured
  - Vascular changes occur due to release of mediators from adjacent tissue

DEPTH OF INJURY

- Superficial (first degree)
  - Involves only superficial epidermis
  - Example: sunburn

- Signs and symptoms
  - Pain, dry, redness, blanches with pressure, no tissue or nerve damage
- Healing time, 3–5 days
- Partial thickness (second degree)
  - Involves epidermis and varying amounts of dermis
    - Some dermis: superficial partial thickness
      - Signs and symptoms
        - Blisters form within minutes, blanches with pressure, bright red to pale ivory in color, appears moist
      - Healing time 7–21 days
    - Lower dermis to subcutaneous tissue: deep partial thickness
      - Example: scald burn
      - Signs and symptoms
        - Pain, mottled, waxy, dry or moist
      - Healing time 30 days to several months
- Full thickness: (third degree)
  - Destruction of epidermis and dermis
  - Involves underlying tissue: subcutaneous adipose tissue, fascia, muscle, bone
  - Example: flame burn
  - Involves loss of massive amounts of body fluids
  - Signs and symptoms
    - Absence of pain; white, red, or charred skin; edematous skin; dry, leathery, inelastic; no blanching
  - High risk for hypovolemic shock and infection
  - Requires skin grafting

TOTAL BODY SURFACE AREA (TBSA)

- Palm estimation
  - A child's palm represents approximately 1% of his or her TBSA
  - Useful for estimating scattered burns

- Rule of nines (see Fig. 3–1)
  - Body is divided into multiples of nine that total 100% TBSA
  - Useful in emergent assessment
- Modified Lund and Browder chart
  - *Most accurate* method to determine TBSA in a child
  - Relates age of patient to body surface

EMERGENCY DEPARTMENT (ED) TREATMENT

- Obtain focused history
  - Time of burn injury
  - Mechanism of burn
  - Location of injury
    - Enclosed area versus open area
    - Percent of body surface area (BSA) burned
    - Anatomic location of burns
    - Associated injuries
    - Medications, allergies, past medical history
    - Weight
    - Prehospital treatment
- Airway, breathing, and circulation (ABCs)
  - Airway—assess patency
    - Observe for swelling of airway, foreign body, secretions, stridor, hoarseness
    - Suction as needed
    - Position—elevate head of bed
    - Secure airway: nasotracheal or endotracheal intubation
  - Breathing—assess breathing effectiveness, presence of spontaneous respirations
    - Observe for signs of inhalation injury (see "Inhalation Injury")
    - Provide 100% humidified oxygen
    - Assist with intubation, bronchoscopy
    - Obtain arterial blood gases (ABGs)
    - Monitor pulse oximetry
    - Consider escharotomy for circumferential, full-thickness burns of neck, chest, or abdomen

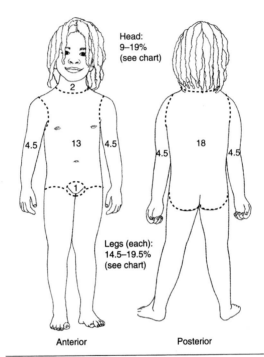

Figure 3–1. Calculating total body surface area (TBSA) burned in children. The standard "rule of nines" and standard body surface charts must be adapted because of the difference in body proportions between adults and children (see text). (Child Burn Size Estimation Table reprinted from Lund, C. C., & Browder, N. C. [1944]. Estimation of burn size. *Surgery, Gynecology, and Obstetrics, 79,* 352–358. By permission of *Surgery, Gynecology, and Obstetrics,* now known as the *Journal of the American College of Surgeons.*)

Child Burn Size Estimation Table
(percent total body surface area)

Burn area	Age (years)				
	1	1–4	5–9	10–14	15
Head	19	17	13	11	9
Neck	2	2	2	2	2
Anterior trunk	13	13	13	13	13
Posterior trunk	18	18	18	18	18
Genitalia	1	1	1	1	1
Upper extremity (each)	9	9	9	9	9
Lower extremity (each)	14.5	15.5	17.5	18.5	19.5

Modified Lund and Browder Chart (TBSA [%])

Burned Area	Age (yr)					
	1	1–4	5–9	10–14	15	Adult
Head	19	17	13	11	9	7
Neck	2	2	2	2	2	3
Anterior trunk	13	13	13	13	13	13
Posterior trunk	13	13	13	13	13	13
Right buttock	2.5	2.5	2.5	2.5	2.5	2.5
Left buttock	2.5	2.5	2.5	2.5	2.5	2.5
Genitalia	1	1	1	1	1	1
Right upper arm	4	4	4	4	4	4
Left upper arm	4	4	4	4	4	4
Right lower arm	3	3	3	3	3	3
Left lower arm	3	3	3	3	3	3
Right hand	2.5	2.5	2.5	2.5	2.5	2.5
Left hand	2.5	2.5	2.5	2.5	2.5	2.5
Right thigh	5.5	6.5	8	8.5	9	9.5
Left thigh	5.5	6.5	8	8.5	9	9.5
Right leg	5	5	5.5	6	6.5	7
Left leg	5	5	5.5	6	6.5	7
Right foot	3.5	3.5	3.5	3.5	3.5	3.5
Left foot	3.5	3.5	3.5	3.5	3.5	3.5

From Emergency Nurses Association: Trauma Nursing Core Course Instructor Manual, 4th ed. Park Ridge, IL, ENA, 1995, p. 268.

Fluid Replacement Formulas (guide to determine rate of fluid replacement)

Time	Solution	Parkland Formula	Brooke Formula
First 24 hr	Crystalloid	4 mL/kg/% burn	1.5 mL/kg/% burn
	Colloid	None	0.5 mL/kg/% burn
	Dextrose and water	None	2000 mL
Second 24 hr	Crystalloid	None	0.75–1.125 mL/kg/% burn
	Colloid	0–2000 mL	0.25–0.375 mL/kg/% burn
	Dextrose and water	2–4000 mL	2000 mL

- Assisted/mechanical ventilation as required
- Circulation—assess effectiveness of circulation
  - Excess catecholamine release may affect heart rate and blood pressure
    - Evaluate volume status by renal perfusion
  - IV access immediately: preferred site, unburned upper extremity
    - Two large-bore access sites
    - Obtain laboratory specimens with venipuncture
      - Complete blood count with differential, electrolytes, glucose, blood urea nitrogen, creatinine
      - Carbon monoxide (CO) level
      - Blood type and screen
      - Clotting studies
      - Toxicology screen, as indicated
    - Administer warmed IV fluids
    - See "Fluid Replacement"
  - Inotropes may be necessary for children with >30–40% BSA burn
    - Dopamine, dobutamine
  - Assess neurovascular status distal to burn
  - Obtain 12-lead electrocardiogram in all electrical burns
- Other interventions
  - Urinary catheterization
    - Urinalysis
    - Urine pigmentation may indicate
      - Red blood cell (RBC) damage, release of hemoglobin, muscle damage, release of myoglobin
  - Gastric intubation
    - Decrease gastric distention from ileus
    - Prevent vomiting
    - Administer antacids
    - Use tracheostomy tape rather than adhesive tape to secure
- Monitor patient response

- Urinary output >1 mL/kg/hr
- Stop the burning process
  - Remove all clothing and jewelry
  - Cool water (never ice) soaks to burn areas
  - Maintain body temperature—normothermia
- Pain control
  - Elevate and cover burn wounds
  - Administer IV analgesics, sedatives
    - Give IV route (IM absorption may be compromised)
    - Morphine sulfate 0.1–0.2 mg/kg/dose slow IV push
    - Meperidine (Demerol) 1.0–1.5 mg/kg/dose slow IV push
    - Midazolam (Versed) 0.08 mg/kg/dose slow IV push
    - Assess effectiveness of pain control frequently
  - Avoid narcotics if patient has head injury
- Tetanus prophylaxis
- Burn wound care
  - Discuss with burn center staff
  - Remove superficial debris (dirt, foreign objects)
  - Minor to moderate burns
    - Cleanse burned areas
    - Débride broken blisters
    - Apply topical antibiotics
      - 1% silver sulfadiazine—most common
      - Antibiotic ointments (e.g., neomycin, bacitracin, Polysporin) for face, leave uncovered
      - Instruct family to change dressing every 24 hr
  - Moderate to severe burns
    - See "Guidelines for Transfer to a Burn Center"
    - Apply dry sterile dressings prior to transfer
- Maintain high index of suspicion for child maltreatment when history and burn injury is inconsistent

FLUID REPLACEMENT

- Fluid replacement is calculated from time of burn injury
- Up to 50% TBSA is considered
  - Replacement of fluids for >50% TBSA burn may result in overhydration
- For the first 24 hours
  - Administer ½ total amount of fluid in first 8 hr
  - Administer ¼ total amount of fluid in second 8 hr
  - Administer ¼ total amount of fluid in third 8 hr
- Fluid resuscitation may be adequate if
  - Urine output is >1 mL/kg/hr
  - Normothermic
  - Normotensive
- Calculations for fluid replacement based on weight, percent of TBSA burn, and other injuries
- Indications
  - Significant electrical burns
  - Partial-thickness or deeper burns
    - >10% TBSA in children
- Objectives
  - Replace plasma volume
  - Maintain tissue perfusion
  - Limit edema
- Colloid replacement
  - Used at 8–24 hr after burn injury as capillary permeability changes begin to reverse
    - Albumin (or fresh frozen plasma if child has coagulation abnormalities)
- Lactated Ringer's solution is fluid of choice
  - Isotonic, similar to extracellular fluid
- Monitor glucose in young children
- Patients at risk for altered fluid needs
  - Preexisting cardiac or renal disease, inhalation injury, diabetes, electrical injury, burns >80% BSA
  - Consider monitoring central venous pressure, pulmonary capillary wedge pressures

- Monitor for development of pulmonary edema
- Monitor vital signs

GUIDELINES FOR TRANSFER TO A BURN CENTER

- Partial-thickness and full-thickness burns >10% TBSA in patients <10 yr
- Partial-thickness and full-thickness burns >20% TBSA in other age groups
- Deep partial-thickness and full-thickness burns that threaten function/cosmetics
  - Face, genitalia, hands, perineum, feet, major joints
- Full-thickness burns >5% TBSA, any age
- Significant electrical burns (includes lightning injury)
- Chemical burns that threaten function/cosmetics
- Inhalation injury
- Circumferential burns of extremity or chest
- Burn injury in patients with preexisting medical disorders that could complicate management, prolong recovery, or affect mortality
  - Diabetes, heart disease, respiratory disease
- Burn injury with concomitant trauma
- Hospitals without qualified personnel or equipment for the care of children
- Burn injury in children who will require social/emotional and/or long-term rehabilitative support, including cases involving suspected child maltreatment

Inhalation Injury

- Most common killer in fires
- Inhalation of smoke and other toxins leads to tracheobronchitis
- Inhalation of heat causes upper airway damage

SIGNS AND SYMPTOMS

- Primary manifestation of smoke inhalation is lower airway injury, which may not be evident for 24–48 hr
- High index of suspicion if the following are present
  - Lower airway distress; i.e., wheezing
  - Facial, neck, torso burns
  - Singed nasal hairs
  - "Burning" discomfort in throat or chest
  - Carbonaceous sputum
- Important considerations
  - Length of exposure
  - Area of exposure (open versus enclosed space)
  - Type of material burned

ED DIAGNOSIS AND INTERVENTIONS

- Fiberoptic bronchoscopy is "gold standard" for diagnosing lower airway injury
- Xenon scan within 48 hr of injury may demonstrate areas of decreased gas washout consistent with airway obstruction
- Provide 100% FIO_2
- Intubate as indicated for high-risk patient (Table 3–1)
- High-risk patients should be intubated immediately, whereas low-risk patients should be observed closely

COMPLICATIONS OF INHALATION INJURY

- Assess for
  - Upper airway edema, hoarseness, stridor, dysphagia
  - Atelectasis, tachypnea, hypoxemia, decreased P_{CO_2}, dyspnea
  - Interstitial edema, pulmonary crackles, tachycardia, cough productive of frothy pink sputum

Table 3–1. Intubation

High Risk	Low Risk
Decreased level of consciousness	Small superficial facial burns
Deep burns to face and neck	Carbonaceous sputum
Edema/sloughing of mucosa in upper airway	Increased respiratory rate
	Wheezes on auscultation
Stridor, hoarseness	Absence of slough of mucosa in upper airway
Supraclavicular retractions	Satisfactory ABGs
Respiratory distress (Pao_2 <60 mm Hg; Pco_2 >55 mm Hg)	

From Singh NC: Manual of Pediatric Critical Care. Philadelphia, W.B. Saunders, 1997, p. 296.

- Bronchitis, frequent cough, dyspnea
- Pneumonia, fever, chills, cough productive of purulent sputum, chest pain
- Respiratory distress, increased respiratory effort, tachypnea, hypoxemia, elevated Pco_2
- When to suspect CO poisoning
  - History reveals an enclosed space burn, and/or pets in the home were found dead without obvious cause
  - Carboxyhemoglobin levels >10%
  - Change in level of consciousness
  - Cherry-red skin color
  - Headache, dizziness, nausea
  - Tachycardia, tachypnea
  - ED interventions
    - Administer 100% FIO_2
    - Consider intubation to support respirations in patients with decreased level of consciousness
    - Consider hyperbaric oxygen if CO levels >30–40%

HEAT EMERGENCIES

- Factors affecting the body's ability to maintain normothermia

- Drugs/medications
- Strenuous activity
- High ambient temperatures/humidity
- Age
- Clothing
- Illness/injury

Heat Cramps

- Those especially at risk include
  - Children involved in athletics
  - Chronically ill children
  - Very young children when the air temperature is greater than the skin temperature
- Heat cramps are the result of overworked, fatigued muscles (especially shoulders, thighs, calves, abdomen)
- Often associated with
  - Ingestion of large amounts of hypotonic fluids (water) during or after exertion
  - Profuse sweating without salt replacement
  - High environmental temperature and low humidity

SIGNS AND SYMPTOMS

- Muscle cramps, especially legs
- Nausea
- Tachycardia
- Pallor
- Diaphoresis
- Cool skin

ED TREATMENT

- Sodium chloride PO
  - May give oral salt solution of 1 tsp NaCl in 500 mL water. Encourage child to drink 20 mL/kg during 1 hr
- If severe, give NaCl IV at 20 mL/kg over 1–2 hr
- Provide a cool environment
- Rest

Heat Exhaustion

- Heat exhaustion is the result of fluid *and* electrolyte depletion
  - Often occurs over a prolonged period
  - Especially in very young
  - May be associated with high temperature and continuous sweating
  - May be associated with diarrhea

SIGNS AND SYMPTOMS

- Thirst
- Malaise, fatigue
- Muscle cramping
- Headache
- Nausea, vomiting
- Orthostatic hypotension
- Normal (or minimal elevation) body temperature

ED TREATMENT

- Fluids and electrolytes PO or IV
  - 20 mL/kg of 0.9 NaCl IV over 30 min
- Provide a cool environment
- Sprinkle water over child's body to increase evaporative losses
- Rest

Heat Stroke

- Serious, may be life-threatening
- Heat stroke is the result of the body's inability to maintain normothermia
- May be associated with exercise in hot environment
- May be seen in children with cystic fibrosis from excessive sweating and salt loss
- Evidenced by
  - A severe depletion of fluids and electrolytes
  - An increased core temperature

- High core temperatures depress central nervous system (CNS), heart, and cellular function
- Every 1°C (1.8°F) increase in core temperature results in a 13% increase in metabolism

SIGNS AND SYMPTOMS

- Hot, dry skin
- Hyperpyrexia >40°C (104°F)
- Tachycardia
- Tachypnea
- Hypotension
- Decreased level of consciousness, confusion, disorientation
- May progress to coma and posturing

ED TREATMENT

- Ensure ABCs
- IV fluid and electrolytes
  - 0.9 NaCl at 20 mL/kg over 30–45min
- Rapid cooling measures
  - Drenching or immersion in cool water
  - Sprinkle child, then fan to speed evaporative losses
  - Cooling blankets
- Chlorpromazine (Thorazine) or diazepam (Valium) may be indicated to control shivering
- Insertion of urinary catheter to monitor output/fluid status
- Insertion of gastric tube

COMPLICATIONS OF HEAT STROKE

- Acute tubular necrosis (ATN)
- Dysrhythmias
- Rhabdomyolysis
- Myoglobinuria
- Disseminated intravascular coagulation (DIC)

COLD-RELATED EMERGENCIES

Frostbite

- Occurs in body parts exposed to prolonged freezing temperatures and wet environment
- Ice crystals form and expand in extracellular spaces if tissue temperature <15°C (59°F)
  - Cell membranes rupture
  - Histamine release
  - Increased capillary membrane permeability
  - RBC aggregation
  - Microvascular occlusion
- The goal of treating frostbite is to protect immediately surrounding areas
- Frostbite is often accompanied by hypothermia

SUPERFICIAL

Signs and Symptoms
- Extends to subcutaneous tissue
- No blanching when pressure is applied to area
- Tissue soft
- Usual sites: nose, ears, cheeks, toes, fingertips
- Burning, tingling, numbness in area

ED Treatment
- Warm water soaks, maintain constant water temperature 40–43°C (104–110°F)
- Do not rub area
- Area will be painful, flushed, edematous after it thaws
- Keep warm with clean dry coverings

DEEP

Signs and Symptoms
- Extends to below subcutaneous tissue
- Tissue firm, unable to depress
- Previously frostbitten areas are at higher risk

- Skin white, waxy
- Child describes burning pain, warmth, then numbness with edema

ED Treatment
- Handle injured part gently while removing all clothing
- Do not rub area
- Prevent further heat loss
- Protect area from injury
- Administer analgesics
- Administer tetanus prophylaxis as indicated
- Antibiotics may be indicated
- Warm water soaks, maintain constant temperature: 40–43°C (104–110°F) for 20–30 min
- After thawing, area may be bluish in color, may remain swollen; blisters may appear in 1–7 days; gangrene may develop later
- Escharotomy may be indicated in presence of vascular constriction
- May discharge to home when skin becomes pliable and erythematous
- Encourage warmed oral fluids

Hypothermia (Table 3–2)

- Use hypothermia thermometer to measure core body temperature
  - If <35°C (95°F) hypothermia exists
- Hypothermia is both a symptom and a clinical disease
- Body is unable to maintain normothermia

CONTRIBUTING FACTORS

- Very young age
- Extreme exposure, submersion injury
- Poor health and nutritional status
- Various medications, drugs

Table 3-2. Hypothermia

Category	Temperature	Signs and Symptoms	ED Treatment
Mild	35–36°C 93–95°F	Conscious, alert Shivering Decreased coordination Slurred speech Amnesia	Warm water bath: 40–43°C (104–110°F) Warm PO fluids of glucose/sugar solutions Avoid caffeine Warm blankets; heating blankets, warm packs Increase room temperature
Moderate	30–34°C 86–93°F	Difficulty speaking Absence of shivering Muscular rigidity Hyperglycemia Decrease in heart and respiratory rates, blood pressure Atrial arrhythmias	Ensure ABCs Provide 100% oxygen Monitor pulse oximetry Obtain ABGs Monitor cardiac rhythm, urine output, core temperature Administer warmed crystalloid IV fluids at 45°C (avoid lactated Ringer's solution)

| Severe | <30°C
<86°F | Unconscious
Erratic, weak to absent pulse and heart tones
Significant hypotension
Erratic, shallow respirations to apnea
Ventricular arrythmias (ventricular fibrillation to asystole)
Cardiopulmonary arrest | *Initiate active core rewarming*
Heated humidified oxygen by mask or ventilator (ventilator should be warmed to 40–45°C)
Gastric, bladder, or colonic lavage with warmed fluids at 45°C
Peritoneal lavage with 10–20 mL/kg potassium-free crystalloid dialysate at 45°C
Hemodialysis or cardiopulmonary bypass
Increase core temperature 10–12°C/hr |

Adapted from Tipsord-Klinkhammer B, Andreoni CP: Quick Reference for Emergency Nursing. Philadelphia, W.B. Saunders, 1998, pp. 70–71.

AT CORE TEMPERATURE <28°C (82.4°F), THERMOREGULATION IS LOST

- Resulting in
  - Vasodilation
  - Impaired cardiac and CNS function
  - Slowed nerve conduction
  - Cardiac irritability
- At this temperature, pharmacologic and electrical interventions are usually not effective
- Rewarming is the priority
- Avoid discontinuation of resuscitation measures until core temperature is 32°C (90°F)
- Avoid rewarming shock
  - Shock symptoms are due to initial vasodilation
  - Peripheral areas are rewarmed faster than the core
  - Lactic acid is released and shunted to the heart

Selected Bibliography

Barkin RM, Rosen P: Emergency Pediatrics: A Guide to Ambulatory Care, 4th ed. St. Louis, Mosby–Year Book, 1994.

Broyles BE: Clinical Companion for Ashwill and Droske Nursing Care of Children: Principles and Practice. Philadelphia, W.B. Saunders, 1997.

Shriners Burn Hospital: Information for the Referral of Pediatric Burn Patients. Cincinnati, Shriners Burn Hospital, 1997.

Singh N: Manual of Pediatric Critical Care. Philadelphia, W.B. Saunders, 1997.

Soud TE, Rogers JS: Manual of Pediatric Emergency Nursing. St. Louis, Mosby–Year Book, 1998.

Tipsord-Klinkhammer B, Andreoni C: Quick Reference for Emergency Nursing. Philadelphia, W.B. Saunders, 1998.

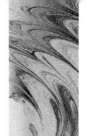

Chapter 4
Eye, Ear, Nose, and Throat

FOREIGN BODY

- Self-insertion of small objects, such as rocks, beads, vegetable matter, small batteries into ears or nose
- Insects crawling or flying into the ear canal (e.g., cockroaches, mosquitoes, beetles, flies)
- Generally can visualize the object or insect with otoscope and/or nasal speculum
- Common in preschool-age children

Signs and Symptoms

- May be asymptomatic, or may have signs and symptoms of an infection
- Organic matter may break down or germinate
  - Purulent or foul-smelling discharge from ear or nostril common with organic matter
- Generally unilateral origin
- May have ear pain or nasal pain, depending on insertion site
- Possible fever
- May exhibit concomitant otitis, sinusitis, or conjunctivitis
- If insect is present, child may verbalize buzzing, flapping, or crawling sensation
  - Smaller child may cry, pull or swat at ear

Emergency Department (ED) Treatment

- Irrigate the ear with warm tapwater or saline
  - Never use cold water as an irrigant for for-

eign body removal, as it may stimulate vomiting

- Do not use water for ear irrigation if vegetable matter is suspected or confirmed
  - Causes vegetable matter to absorb water and expand
- Instillation of 2% lidocaine (Xylocaine) solution or alcohol into ear canal containing a live insect may stun or kill it
  - May use mineral oil, but this may make insect removal slightly more difficult due to oily texture
- For ear irrigation, use a standard ear syringe, commercial irrigation set, or 20- to 30-cc syringe with an IV angiocatheter (shortened and the stylet removed)
- Nasal foreign bodies generally removable with forceps (e.g., bayonet) or suction
- Adequately restrain child to prevent injury or inadvertent pushing of the foreign body further into the orifice
  - Papoose or wrap child in a sheet
- Consider conscious sedation or ear, nose, and throat (ENT) consultation

OTITIS MEDIA

- Infection of the middle ear
- A common cause of fever in children ages 6 mo–2 yr and ages 4–6 yr
  - Coincides with entry into preschool or kindergarten
- Caused by a variety of organisms, both bacterial and viral
  - *Streptococcus pneumoniae, Haemophilus influenzae, Streptococcus pyogenes, Moraxella catarrhalis*, and *Staphylococcus aureus* are common causative agents
- Can also be caused by effusion, barotrauma, or trauma to the tympanic membrane (TM)

Complications of Untreated Otitis Media

- Hearing loss
- Abscess (neck or intracranial)
- Mastoiditis
- Meningitis
- TM rupture

Signs and Symptoms

- Ear pain verbalized by older child, or pulling at ear by nonverbal child
- Fever
- Loss of appetite
- Fussiness in small child

ED Treatment

- Antibiotics
- Analgesics
- Antipyretics
- Thorough discharge instructions to caregiver
  - Discourage bottles in bed and encourage upright feedings
    - Negative pressure in eustachian tubes may draw feeding (e.g., formula) into ear
  - Nonsmoking environment for child
    - Smoking around children increases nasal congestion and results in obstruction of middle ear drainage
- Recheck at end of antibiotics

EXTERNAL OTITIS

- Infection or inflammation of the external ear
- Sometimes called swimmer's ear
- More common in older children

Causes

- Gram-negative organisms
- Fungi
- Dermatosis

Signs and Symptoms

- Swollen ear canal
- Drainage or crusting
- Pruritic ear
- Muffled hearing
- Possible full sensation or feeling as if water were in ear
- Tugging or pulling at ear
- Fussiness

ED Treatment

- Anti-inflammatory otic solutions
- Use of an ear wick is often necessary to instill medications into the swollen ear canal
- Analgesic drops as needed for pain
- Instructions to caregiver for no swimming or immersion of ear into water
  - May require ear plugs in the future during swimming or bathing

CONJUNCTIVITIS

- Inflammation of the conjunctiva
  - Thin lining of the posterior eyelid and the eyeball (except the cornea)
- Variety of causal agents
  - Bacterial
    - Most common cause in children
  - Viral
  - Allergic
  - From foreign body
- Ophthalmia neonatorum
  - From chemical irritation (silver nitrate instillation after birth) or maternal sexually transmitted disease
    - Chlamydia is most common infectious agent
    - *Neisseria gonorrhoeae*
- Recurrent conjunctivitis in infants may indicate a nasolacrimal duct obstruction

- Complications of conjunctivitis are rare except when the cornea is involved
  - May lead to permanent blindness from scarring, perforations, or tissue death

Signs and Symptoms

- "Pink eye"
- Drainage serous to purulent
  - Crusting of eyelids common in children
- Swollen eyelids
- Pruritus
- Pain
- Tearing
- Generally bilateral unless caused by a foreign body

ED Treatment

- Visual acuity if child is able to identify shapes or read
- Topical antibiotic ointment or drops to prevent a superinfection
- Parental or caregiver instructions
  - Warm compresses to eyes
  - Medications as directed until no drainage for 48 hr
  - Frequent hand washing
  - Measures to avoid cross contamination from one eye to the other
    - No towel or facial cloth sharing
    - Wipe from the inner canthus downward and outward away from the opposite eye
  - Avoid rubbing the eyes

PERIORBITAL CELLULITIS

- Infection of the tissues surrounding the eye
- Potentially life-threatening conditions may result
  - Cavernous sinus thrombosis
  - Intracranial infection

- Meningitis
- Septicemia
- Vision loss may occur if treatment is delayed
- Can affect both small children (ages 2–4 yr) and older children and adolescents

Signs and Symptoms

- Fever
- Periorbital swelling and erythema
- Pain
- Symptoms progress rapidly

ED Treatment

- Airway, breathing, and circulation (ABCs)
- Visual acuity if child is able to identify shapes or read
- Complete blood count (CBC) and consider blood cultures
- Computed tomography scan to determine existence of orbital, intracranial, or sinus involvement
- IV access if indicated
  - IV antibiotics as indicated
- May require a lumbar puncture to rule out meningitis
- Preparation for hospital admission unless case is mild
  - Discharge instructions to parents or caregiver
    - Antibiotic therapy (may last as long as 2–3 wk)
    - Return for medical care as scheduled or if pain, fever develop

EPISTAXIS

- Bleeding from the nose
  - Generally unilateral
- Common in childhood
- Variety of causes

- Picking of nose
- Blunt trauma
- Mucosal inflammation (allergic rhinitis or upper respiratory infection [URI])
- Foreign body
- Forceful blowing of nose
- Clotting factor disorders
  - Hemophilia
  - Von Willebrand's disease
- Vascular abnormalities
  - Leukemia
  - Thrombocytopenia
- Kiesselbach's triangle common site of anterior epistaxis
  - A thin, highly vascular area of the nasal septum that receives its blood supply from the internal and external carotid artery system

Signs and Symptoms

- Blood from nostril(s)
  - Anterior bleed usually resolvable with direct pressure
  - Posterior bleed generally more profuse and harder to control
- Severe blood loss is uncommon, but can occur
  - Pale color
  - Signs of hypovolemia

ED Treatment

- ABCs
- Direct pressure to area
  - Noseclips are helpful
- Topical vasoconstrictors or anesthetics (4% cocaine solution; 4% lidocaine (Xylocaine) or tetracaine with epinephrine)
- Topical thrombin
- Cautery
  - Silver nitrate
- Packing if indicated (rare in children)

- Petrolatum gauze or cellulose tampon
- Hemostatic material such as Gelfoam
- Nasal balloon catheters
- If hypovolemia suspected
  - CBC, type and cross-match, coagulation studies
  - IV access
- Instructions to parents or caregivers to include
  - Prevent picking of nose by applying mittens or socks to hands
  - Cool mist humidifier for nighttime or naptime use
  - Bleeding control measures
    - Return for medical care if bleeding is not controlled after 20 min
  - Avoid aspirin use

SINUSITIS

- Inflammation of one or more of the paranasal sinuses
  - Frontal and maxillary sinuses are palpable during examination
  - Ethmoid sinuses are most frequently affected in children <10 yr
- Infection results from obstruction of secretions from the sinuses
  - Stagnation of secretions promotes growth of bacteria or fungi
- Infections can be acute or chronic
- Chronic sinusitis contributing factors
  - Cigarette smoke (passive in nonsmoking children; active in smoking adolescents)
  - Air pollution
  - Inhalation of street drugs such as cocaine or heroin
- Complications of chronic or partially treated sinusitis
  - Meningitis
  - Orbital abscess
  - Cavernous sinus thrombosis

- Brain abscess
- Osteomyelitis of the maxillary or frontal bones
- Mucocele
  - A cystic structure filled with mucus

Signs and Symptoms

- Purulent nasal discharge
- Cough (worse at night)
- Fever
- Facial pain (if able to verbalize)
- Periorbital swelling
- Malodorous breath

ED Treatment

- Based on symptoms
- Sinus x-rays in older children (>5 yr) may show
  - Air-fluid levels
  - Sinus opacification
  - Bone destruction in a chronic state
- Antibiotic therapy
  - Amoxicillin is the drug of choice
  - Child should respond to therapy within 72 hr
  - Decongestants
  - Antihistamines
  - Antipyretics
- Instructions to parents or caregiver
  - Nonsmoking environment
  - Humidifier for nighttime use or naptime use
  - Return if the child develops redness or swelling of the periorbital area

PHARYNGITIS

- Inflammation of the musculomembranous tube situated at the back of the nose, mouth, and larynx
  - Also known as "sore throat"
- Uncommon in children <12 mo

- Peak occurrence between ages 4 and 7 yr
- Caused by
  - Viral agents
  - Bacterial agents
    - Group A beta-hemolytic streptococcus is most common
      - Prevalence for this type of infection is late winter and early spring
      - Can trigger rheumatic fever or glomerulo-nephritis
    - Gonococcus
      - Suspect sexual abuse in children
        - Gonococcal pharyngitis is not uncommon in the sexually active adolescent

Signs and Symptoms

- Throat pain (if able to verbalize)
  - Fussiness in nonverbal child
- URI symptoms
- Fever
- Cough
- Malaise as exhibited by decreased activity or play

ED Treatment

- Based on symptoms
- Antipyretics
- Rapid strep screen
  - Throat culture if rapid strep screen is negative
- Antibiotics if screen is positive
  - Penicillin is the antibiotic of choice
    - Erythromycin if allergy to penicillin
- Instructions to parents or caregiver
  - Warm salt water gargles in older children
  - Complete the course of antibiotics
  - Soft diet with plenty of liquids

TONSILLITIS

- Inflammation of the tonsils
  - Palatine or faucial tonsils located on each side of the oropharynx
  - Pharyngeal tonsils or adenoids located in the posterior wall of the nasopharynx
  - Lingual tonsils located at the base of the tongue
  - Tubal tonsils located near the posterior nasopharyngeal opening of the eustachian tubes
- Tonsils have a filtering function that protects the respiratory and GI tracts
- Infections result from
  - Viral agents
  - Bacterial agents
    - Group A beta-hemolytic streptococcus is most common
  - Fungi
- May be acute, chronic, or recurring
- Tonsils can become cryptic (with concealed pockets)
  - Foreign bodies can become embedded in the crypts
    - Fingernails
    - Seeds
    - Fishbones
- Complication is a tonsillar abscess
  - An abscess forming around one or both tonsils
  - Also known as "quinsy"

Signs and Symptoms

- Throat pain (if able to verbalize)
  - Fussiness in nonverbal child
    - Tonsillitis is uncommon in children <1 yr
- Enlarged tonsils
- URI symptoms
- Fever
- Cough

- Malaise, as exhibited by decreased activity or play
- Abscess characterized by previously cited signs plus
  - Edema of posterior pharynx
    - Causes a muffled voice
  - Dysphagia or drooling
  - Pus on the tonsil(s)
  - May be unilateral or bilateral

ED Treatment

- Based on symptoms
- Antipyretics
- Rapid strep screen
  - Throat culture if rapid strep screen is negative
- Antibiotics if screen is positive
  - Penicillin is the antibiotic of choice
    - Erythromycin if allergy to penicillin
- Follow-up with primary care provider for possible tonsillectomy
  - Rarely performed on children <4 yr
  - Indicated only for massive hypertrophy of the palatine tonsils
- If tonsillar abscess
  - ABCs, with continuous assessment of airway patency
  - Emergency airway equipment readily available
  - IV access
    - IV antibiotics
    - IV hydration if indicated
  - Preparation for aspiration of the abscess if indicated
- Instructions to parents or caregiver for tonsillitis
  - Warm salt water gargles in older children
  - Complete the course of antibiotics
  - Soft diet with plenty of liquids
  - Do not share eating utensils, drinking glasses, or toothbrushes

UVULITIS

- An inflammation of the uvula
  - The conical appendix hanging from the free edge of the soft palate
    - Contains the uvular muscle
      - Covered by a mucous membrane
- Can occasionally swell
- Very rare in infants
- Can be caused by
  - Viral agents
  - Bacterial agents
    - Group A beta-hemolytic streptococcus is most common
  - Fungi

Signs and Symptoms

- Swollen uvula on inspection
  - Child may describe as "something is hanging in my throat" (if verbal)
- Sore throat
- Dysphagia

ED Treatment

- Generally self-limiting and does not require treatment unless a positive screen for group A beta-hemolytic streptococcus
- Antibiotics if strep screen is positive

Chapter 5
Fluids and Electrolytes

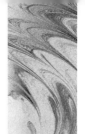

IMBALANCES

- The body is primarily composed of fluid (water and solutes)
  - Intracellular fluid (ICF) (Table 5–1)
  - Extracellular fluid (ECF)
    - Intravascular (plasma)
    - Interstitial fluid (IF)
    - Transcellular (cerebrospinal fluid, sweat, synovial, pericardial, and gastrointestinal [GI] secretions)
- Infants and children are most susceptible to fluid and electrolyte imbalances
  - The younger the child, the greater the susceptibility to fluid and electrolyte disturbances with illness, trauma, or fever
  - Higher metabolic rates
    - A turnover of water relative to the total body water is more rapid
- Two types of water loss
  - Sensible water loss
    - Urine and normal bowel movements

Age Group	Intracellular Fluid (%)	Extracellular Fluid (%)
Table 5–1. Percent Body Weight of Intracellular vs. Extracellular Fluid		
Infants	35	40
Children to ages 3–5 yr	34	30
Adolescents	30	20

- Insensible water loss
  - Skin
    - Perspiration
  - Respiration
    - Rapid respiratory rates in infants and children, especially with fever, can increase evaporative water loss
- Dehydration can result from
  - Reduced fluid intake
  - Increased fluid losses
  - Continuing normal losses
  - A combination of all of the above
- Loss of body weight >1%/day represents loss of body water
- Electrolytes make up majority of body's solutes
  - Primary electrolytes are (Table 5–2)
    - Sodium (Na)
    - Potassium (K)
    - Chloride (Cl)
    - Calcium (Ca)

HYPONATREMIA (DECREASED BLOOD SODIUM)

- Usually means excess body water rather than total body sodium

Table 5–2. Normal Serum Electrolyte Values for the Pediatric Patient

Age Group	Sodium (mEq/L)	Potassium (mEq/L)	Chloride (mEq/L)	Total Calcium (mg/dL)
Newborn (cord blood)	116–166	5.6–12.0	96–106	8.2–11.2
Infant	139–146	4.1–5.3	96–106	7.6–10.4
Child	138–145	3.4–4.7	97–107	8.8–10.8

Modified from Chernecky C, Berger B: Laboratory Tests and Diagnostic Procedures, 2nd ed. Philadelphia, W.B. Saunders, 1997, pp. 351, 470.

- Conditions associated with hyponatremia
  - Severe burns
  - Severe diarrhea
  - Vomiting
  - Malabsorption syndrome
  - Diabetic ketoacidosis
  - Severe nephritis
  - Cystic fibrosis
  - Cerebral palsy
  - Head trauma
  - Salicylate toxicity
  - Water intoxication (can occur as a result of excessive tapwater in formula or to drink)
  - Syndrome of inappropriate antidiuretic hormone (SIADH) secretion

Signs and Symptoms

- Lethargy
- Behavioral changes
- Anorexia or poor feeding
- Tachycardia
- Hypotension
- Abdominal and other muscle cramps
- Headache
- Seizures

HYPERNATREMIA (INCREASED BLOOD SODIUM)

- May be caused by several factors
  - Increased insensible water loss
  - Insufficient antidiuretic hormone (ADH) production
  - Reduced renal response to ADH
  - Hypodipsia
  - Salt poisoning

Conditions Associated With Hypernatremia

- Gastroenteritis
- Hypovolemia

- Salicylate toxicity
- Diabetes insipidus

Signs and Symptoms

- Dehydration
- Weight loss
- Tachycardia
- Hypotension
- Thirst
- Decreased urine output
  - Number of wet diapers is decreased
- Nausea and/or vomiting
- Agitation

HYPOKALEMIA (POTASSIUM DEFICIENCY)

- Most frequent cause of potassium deficiency is through gastrointestinal loss

Conditions Associated With Hypokalemia

- Cerebral palsy
- Diabetes mellitus
- Gastroenteritis
- Malabsorption syndrome
- Salicylate intoxication
- Starvation
- Stress

Signs and Symptoms

- Malaise
- Thirst
- Anorexia or poor feeding
- Vomiting
- Decreased reflexes
- Depressed T-waves and ventricular ectopy
- Bradycardia or tachycardia

HYPERKALEMIA (INCREASED BLOOD POTASSIUM)

- Most frequent causes of hyperkalemia
  - Renal failure
  - Cell damage (burns, trauma, surgery)
  - Acidosis (drives potassium out of the cells)

Conditions Associated With Hyperkalemia

- Asthma
- Diabetes mellitus with ketoacidosis
- Renal failure
- Sepsis
- Status epilepticus
- SIADH

Signs and Symptoms

- Irritability
- Diarrhea
- Oliguria
- Muscle cramps
- Peaked T-waves
- Ventricular fibrillation or ventricular tachycardia

HYPOCALCEMIA (REDUCED BLOOD CALCIUM)

- Alkalosis can precipitate hypocalcemia
- Neonatal tetany
  - Results from feeding cow's milk to infants <1 mo
  - Phosphate imbalances produce hypocalcemia

Conditions Associated With Hypocalcemia

- Pseudohypocalcemia (reflecton of reduced albumin)

- Hypoparathyroidism
- Chronic renal failure
- Malabsorption
- Diarrhea
- Rickets
- Food fads that result in vitamin D deficiency

Signs and Symptoms

- Convulsions
- Carpopedal spasm (Trousseau's sign)
- Facial spasms (Chvostek's sign)
- Muscle cramps
- Numbness
- Tetany
- ST-segment and QT interval prolongation

HYPERCALCEMIA (EXCESS BLOOD CALCIUM)

- Rare in children

Conditions Associated With Hypercalcemia

- Hyperparathyroidism
- Prolonged immobilization (body casts)
- Food fads resulting in hypervitaminosis D
- Improper preparation of formula
- Milk-alkali syndrome (excessive intake of milk or antacids)
- Respiratory acidosis

Signs and Symptoms

- Constipation
- Lethargy
- Muscle weakness
- Nausea
- Headache
- Stupor to coma
- Bradycardia leading to cardiac arrest

Table 5-3. ABG Values to Determine Acid-Base Balance Disturbances

	Normal Values	Metabolic Acidosis	Metabolic Alkalosis	Respiratory Acidosis	Respiratory Alkalosis
pH	7.35–7.45	<7.35	>7.45	<7.35	>7.45
PaCO$_2$	40–45 mm Hg	<40 mm Hg	>45 mm Hg	>45 mm Hg	<35 mm Hg
PaO$_2$	80–100 mm Hg	Normal to slightly decreased	Decreased	Decreased	Decreased
HCO$_3$	22–26 mEq/L	<22 mEq/L	>26 mEq/L	Normal to slightly increased	Decreased

Table 5–4. Maintenance IV Fluid Rates for Children

Weight	Amount/hr (mL)
1–10 kg	100 mL/kg/24 hr
10–20 kg	1000 mL *plus* 50 mL/kg for each additional kg over 10 (up to 20 kg), administered over 24 hr
≥21 kg	1500 mL *plus* 20 mL/kg for each additional kg over 21, administered over 24 hr

Adapted from Tipsord-Klinkhammer B, Andreoni C: Quick Reference for Emergency Nursing. Philadelphia, W.B. Saunders, 1998, p. 173.

TREATMENT OF FLUID AND ELECTROLYTE IMBALANCE

- ABCs
- Chemistry, complete blood count, urine for specific gravity, osmolality, and urinalysis
  - Normal specific gravity = 1.002–1.030
  - Normal urine osmolality = 275–295 mOsm/kg
- Arterial blood gases (ABGs) to determine acid-base status (Table 5–3)
- Cardiac monitor
- Administer maintenance IV fluids as indicated (Table 5–4)
- Treat underlying cause

Selected Bibliography

Ashwill J, Droske S: Nursing Care of Children: Principles and Practice. Philadelphia, W.B. Saunders, 1997.

Behrman R, Kligman R: Nelson Essentials of Pediatrics, 3rd ed. Philadelphia, W.B. Saunders, 1998.

Betz C, Sowden L: Mosby's Pediatric Nursing Reference, 3rd ed. St. Louis, Mosby–Year Book, 1996.

Chernecky C, Berger B: Laboratory Tests and Diagnostic Procedures, 2nd ed. Philadelphia, W.B. Saunders, 1997.

Kidd P, Sturt P: Mosby's Emergency Nursing Reference. St. Louis, Mosby–Year Book, 1996.

Tipsord-Klinkhammer B, Andreoni C: Quick Reference for Emergency Nursing. Philadelphia, W.B. Saunders, 1998.

Chapter 6
Gastrointestinal

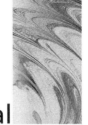

PYLORIC STENOSIS

- Hypertrophy of the pyloric muscle
  - Leads to obstruction at the pyloric sphincter
- Five times more common in male than female live births
  - White infants affected more frequently than black or Asian

Signs and Symptoms

- Projectile vomiting shortly after feeding
  - Vomit ejection of 1–4 ft is hallmark
  - Seen in later stage of disease
- Infant acts chronically hungry
- No evidence of pain
- May fail to gain weight
- Decrease in the amount of stools
- Dehydration signs
  - Dry mucous membranes
  - Decreased tears
  - Decreased voiding
  - Decreased number of wet diapers
  - Sunken fontanel
- Visible epigastric peristaltic waves
- Palpable olive-size mass in right upper quadrant (RUQ) above umbilicus

Emergency Department (ED) Treatment

- Airway, breathing, and circulation (ABCs)
- Complete blood count (CBC), chemistry, urinalysis (UA)
- IV fluid replacement
  - May require potassium administration

- Infusion pump
- Intake and output
- Gastric decompression
  - Nasogastric or orogastric tube insertion

INTUSSUSCEPTION

- Telescoping of one portion of bowel into another
  - Ileocecal valve is most common site
- Occurs between 3 mo and 5 yr
  - Most common age is 3–12 mo
- Cause is unknown but has followed viral illness

Signs and Symptoms

- Sudden, acute, intermittent abdominal pain
  - Draws knees upward
  - Calm, pain-free between episodes
- "Currant jelly" stool is classic sign
  - Stool is mixed with mucus and blood
    - A subsequent normal brown stool indicates a reduction of the intussusception
- Distention of abdomen
- Palpable sausage-like mass in the RUQ
- Dance sign
  - Absence of bowel sound in the right lower quadrant (RLQ)

ED Treatment

- ABCs
- IV access and, if indicated, fluid resuscitation
- CBC, chemistry, consider type and cross-match (T&C)
- Preparation for a barium enema
- Preparation for surgery if previously cited measures are unsuccessful

VOLVULUS

- A twisting of the small intestine
  - Strangulation of superior mesenteric artery
- Results from congenital malrotation of bowel

Signs and Symptoms

- Obstructive signs
  - Acute, constant abdominal pain
  - Distention of the abdomen
  - Vomiting
  - Visible peristaltic waves
- Peritoneal irritation
  - May signal bowel perforation
- Necrosis of intestine results from obstructed blood supply

ED Treatment

- ABCs
- CBC, chemistry, UA, possible T&C
- IV access
  - IV antibiotics if perforation suspected
- Gastric decompression
  - Nasogastric or orogastric tube insertion
- Prepare for surgery as indicated

HIRSCHSPRUNG'S DISEASE

- Aganglionic megacolon
  - Ganglion cells absent, usually in rectum, but can include proximal large colon
  - Four times more common in male than female live births
  - 10–15% affected infants also have Down syndrome
- Abnormal to absent peristaltic activity
  - Results in inability to evacuate bowel
    - Colon dilates and distends

Signs and Symptoms

- Neonate
  - Classic sign is failure to pass meconium within 24–48 hr after birth
  - Vomiting (often bile-stained)
  - Abdominal bloating

- Poor fluid intake by mouth
- Infancy to childhood
  - Failure to thrive
  - Intermittent constipation and diarrhea
  - Enterocolitis signs
    - Watery, explosive diarrhea
    - Fever
  - Abdominal bloating
  - Older children may have chronic constipation
  - Stool described as ribbon-like and malodorous

ED Treatment

- ABCs
- CBC, chemistry
- Abdominal radiographs
- IV access if indicated by electrolyte imbalance
- Long-term treatment includes surgical intervention

MECKEL'S DIVERTICULUM

- Omphalomesenteric fistula
  - Fibrous band that connects the small intestine to the umbilicus
  - Present in 1–3% of total population
    - Twice as common in males than females

Symptoms

- Vague, recurrent abdominal pain
- Can mimic appendicitis
- "Currant jelly" stools (see "Intussusception")

ED Treatment

- ABCs
- CBC, chemistry, T&C if severe bleeding
- Abdominal radiographs
- Nuclear scintigraph (specific)
  - Detects presence of gastric mucosa

VOMITING (see also Gastroenteritis)

- Common in pediatric population
- Persistent vomiting should be diagnosed
- Multiple causes
  - Obstructive
  - Allergic or toxic
  - Infectious (see Gastroenteritis)
  - Central nervous system
  - Psychologic manifestations
- Can quickly lead to dehydration

ED Treatment

- ABCs
- Dependent on cause
- CBC, chemistry
- IV access if indicated for fluid replacement*
  - Assess for dehydration and aggressively treat if present
  - See Table 5–4. Maintenance IV Fluid Rates for Children, and Section VII, Procedure 7 IV Fluid Bolus Administration
- PO fluid replacement (Pedialyte, Infalyte) in small, frequent amounts

DIARRHEA (see also Gastroenteritis)

- Common in pediatric population
  - Diarrhea is not normal and should be diagnosed
- Acute diarrhea
  - A sudden change in frequency/consistency of stools
  - Usually an infectious etiology
  - Can be from food additives or dietary overindulgences
- Chronic diarrhea
  - Multiple causes
    - Problems of motility
    - Malabsorption
    - Allergic or toxic causes

- Anatomic defects
- Inflammatory response long-term in nature
- Increased frequency
- Lasts >2 wk

ED Treatment

- ABCs
- Stool history
  - Number of stools per day or number of soiled diapers
  - Color, consistency, and odor
- CBC, chemistry, stool culture
- IV access if indicated for dehydration*
- See Table 5–4. Maintenance IV Fluid Rates for Children and Section VII, Procedure 7. IV Fluid Bolus Administration
- PO fluids (Pedialyte, Infalyte) in small, frequent amounts

CONSTIPATION

- Passing hard, firm stools
  - Can have bowel movements either regularly or at irregular intervals
- Inability to expel stools, hard or soft
- Wide range of causes
  - Organic
  - Structural
  - Drugs
  - Spinal cord lesions
  - Systemic conditions
  - Mental retardation
  - Diet

Signs and Symptoms

- Abdominal pain
- Nausea and/or vomiting
- Blood-streaked stools
- May have abdominal bloating
- Generally afebrile

ED Treatment

- Stool history
  - Number of stools per day or number of soiled diapers
  - Color, consistency, and odor
- Suppository or enema to induce bowel evacuation
- Parental or caregiver instructions
  - High-fiber diet and increased oral fluid instructions
  - Regular toileting times

GASTROENTERITIS (See Table 6–1)

- Major cause is infectious agent
  - Viral
  - Bacterial
  - Parasitic
- Oral-fecal or person-to-person transmission
- Higher incidence
  - Day-care settings
  - Crowded, unsanitary living conditions
  - Winter months (viral prevalence)
  - Summer months (bacterial prevalence)

Signs and Symptoms

- Diarrhea
- Vomiting
- Abdominal pain
- Fever
- Dehydration
  - Dry mucous membranes
  - Decreased tears
  - Decreased voiding
    - Decreased number of wet diapers
  - Sunken anterior fontanel

ED Treatment

- ABCs
- CBC, chemistry, stool culture

- IV access
  - IV fluid replacement/resuscitation
    - See Table 5–4. Maintenance IV Fluid Rates for Children and Section VII, Procedure 7. IV Fluid Bolus Administration

HEPATITIS (see Table 6–2)

- Inflammation of the liver
- Caused by a variety of viruses
  - Hepatitis A virus (HAV)
  - Hepatitis B virus (HBV)
  - Hepatitis C virus (HCV, non-A, non-B)
  - Hepatitis D virus (HDV, delta virus)
  - Hepatitis E virus (HEV, enteric non-A, non-B)
- Self-limiting or fulminate
- HAV is most common cause/type in children

Signs and Symptoms

- Dependent on causative virus
- Nausea
- Vomiting
- Diarrhea
- RUQ pain
- Malaise
- Fever

Progressive Symptoms

- Jaundiced skin, sclera
- Dark yellow/orange urine
- Paste-colored stools
- Purpura

ED Treatment

- ABCs
- CBC, chemistry, erythrosedimentation rate, UA, prothrombin time (PT), partial thromboplastin time (PTT), and serologic testing
- IV access

Table 6-1. Common Gastroenteritis Causative Agents

Agent	Incubation Period	Description, Transmission (T), and Duration (D)
Rotavirus (viral)	48 hr	Fever, nausea, vomiting; prolonged diarrhea More common in winter (T) Fecal-oral or fecal-respiratory (D) 5-7 days
Adenovirus (viral)	3-10 days	Low-grade fever; watery diarrhea (T) Fecal-oral route (D) 5-12 days
Norwalk virus (viral)	24-48 hr	Nausea, vomiting; fever; general malaise (T) Fecal-oral, droplets, drinking water, food (D) 1-3 days
Escherichia coli (bacterial)	12-72 hr	Perfuse watery diarrhea; fever; vomiting (T) Contaminated feces (D) <3-5 days
Salmonella (bacterial)	6-72 hr	Headache; abdominal pain; nausea and vomiting; diarrhea (T) Ingestion of infected food or feces contaminated food (D) 3-7 days

Organism	Incubation Period	Symptoms / Transmission / Duration
Shigella (bacterial)	1–7 days	Fever; blood, green diarrhea; abdominal pain; nuchal rigidity **(T)** Fecal-oral route **(D)** 7–10 days
Campylobacter (bacterial)	1–10 days	Perfuse watery diarrhea; abdominal pain; fever; nausea and vomiting **(T)** Organism found in food, unpasteurized milk **(D)** 1–4 days
Giardia (protozoan)	5–25 days	Abdominal cramps; diarrhea; steatorrhea; fatigue; can be asymptomatic **(T)** Ingestion of cysts in fecally contaminated water or food **(D)** Variable, can be weeks
Cryptosporidium (parasite)	Not precisely known, but probably ~10 days	Acute diarrhea; common in day care center situations; can cause chronic diarrhea in the immunosuppressed child **(T)** Fecal-oral; animal handlers are at a higher risk of exposure **(D)** 3–14 days

- See Section I, Reference 14. Recommended Childhood Immunization Schedule

APPENDICITIS

- Most common cause of an acute abdomen in children
  - Uncommon in children <2 yr

Signs and Symptoms

- Pain originates in periumbilical area and moves to the RLQ (classic symptom)
- Preferred position is supine with the legs flexed
- Retrocecal appendix presentation may cause right flank pain
- Positive iliopsoas test
  - RLQ pain with passive extension of the hip or with moderate resistance over the thigh as patient flexes right hip
  - Suggestive of inflamed or perforated appendix
- McBurney's point
  - Area of localized pain and rebound tenderness between umbilicus and right iliac crest

Associated Symptoms

- Anorexia
- Nausea, vomiting
- Fever
- Malaise
- Diarrhea or constipation
- Increasing pain with movement

ED Treatment

- ABCs
- CBC, chemistry, UA
- Radiographs (flat and upright abdomen)
- Ultrasound may assist with diagnosis
- IV access

Table 6–2. Hepatitis

Type	Incubation	Description and Transmission (T)
HAV (infectious)	15–50 days	Rapid, acute onset; fever; anorexia; nausea and vomiting (T) Fecal-oral, person-to-person
HBV (serum)	45–180 days	Slower onset; rash; joint pain; jaundice; anorexia (T) Percutaneous or permucosal exposure
HCV (non-A, non-B)	15–160 days	Slower onset; anorexia; nausea and vomiting; jaundice (T) Contaminated blood products, saliva, blood, breast milk, urine, semen
HDV (delta virus)	15–64 days	Only produces infection when HBV is present; can lead to fulminate hepatitis (T) Percutaneous exposure
HEV (enteric non-A, non-B)	14–63 days	Nonchronic, no carrier state (T) Fecal-oral route; contaminated water or poor sanitation

• Preparation for surgery

FOREIGN BODY INGESTION

• Most common in children 6 mo–6 yr
  • Especially during the creeping, crawling, and toddler stages
• Very young children explore environment by putting anything within reach into the mouth
  • Coins
  • Small toys, toy parts, marbles, springs, jacks
  • Buttons
  • Jewelry
  • Dirt and rocks

Signs and Symptoms

• Usually asymptomatic
  • Caregiver may have seen child swallow object
  • Caregiver may suspect ingestion
• Respiratory distress symptoms may be present if esophagus is blocked or pressing on the trachea
  • Wheeze
    • Bilateral if esophagus is blocked or pressing on the trachea
    • Usually unilateral if aspirated into the right or left main stem bronchus
• Stridor
• Use of accessory muscles
• Tachypnea

ED Treatment

• ABCs
• Plain radiograph of GI tract, chest x-ray, neck x-ray as indicated
• Barium swallow if food or radiolucent object
• Preparation for endoscopy or balloon catheter removal if foreign body is lodged in the esophagus

- IV access as indicated
- Conscious sedation as indicated for removal of foreign body
- Disposition is variable
  - Surgery
  - Observation status
  - Home with instructions
    - Check stools for passage of object
    - Return for medical care if pain, vomiting, fever

Chapter 76
Genitourinary

SEXUALLY TRANSMITTED DISEASES (STDs) (Table 7–1)

Categories of Infections

- Bacterial
  - Gonorrhea
  - Chlamydia
  - Syphilis
- Viral
  - Herpes
  - Human papillomavirus (HPV)
  - Hepatitis B virus
  - HIV
- Protozoan
  - Trichomonas
- Fungal
  - Candida

Signs and Symptoms

- Abdominal pain
- Discharge (vaginal/penile)
- Lesions (genital)
- Fever
- Dysuria
- Adolescents can be at greater risk for complications due to delay in seeking medical care
  - Ectopic pregnancy due to scarring
  - HIV risk increased with number of sexual partners

Emergency Department (ED) Treatment and Diagnostic Studies

- Urinalysis (UA), urine pregnancy test, possible urine culture

Table 7–1. Manifestations and Treatment for Sexually Transmitted Diseases

Disease	Incubation	Symptoms	Treatment	Comments
Neisseria gonorrhoeae	3–5 days	Yellow-brown purulent foul-smelling discharge; dysuria in males, may have a milky discharge from penis	Ceftriaxone IM	Also known as drip, whites, strain, GC
Chlamydia trachomatis	5–10 days	None to mucopurulent	Doxycycline, tetracycline, erythromycin	Can be associated with gonorrhea
Trichomonas	7 days	Vaginal itch; frothy green-gray discharge	Metronidazole	Avoid alcohol while taking this drug
Gardnerella vaginalis	5–10 days	Frothy gray-white discharge that smells like fish	Metronidazole	Avoid alcohol while taking this drug
Herpes simplex II	2–12 days	Vesicular lesions; painful urination	Acyclovir	Latent and recurrent phases
HPV (condyloma acuminatum)	Days to months	Warty lesions; often asymptomatic	Topical podophyllin; laser surgery may be indicated in severe cases	Associated with cervical neoplasia
Syphilis	3 wk	Ulcer or chancre; + RPR or + VDRL	Tetracycline, doxycycline, benzathine penicillin	Has primary and secondary stages

RPR, rapid plasma reagin; VDRL, Venereal Disease Research Laboratory (test).

- DNA probe or culture of discharge (male)
- Pelvic examination with DNA probe or cultures (female)
- Potassium hydroxide preparation (slide for yeast)
- Wet mount *(Trichomonas)*
- Medications
  - Instructions not to have sexual contact until all medications are finished
  - Condom instructions and distribution as institutional policy allows
  - Report as indicated to child protection agencies

PELVIC INFLAMMATORY DISEASE (PID)

- Involves pelvic structures
  - Cervix
  - Uterus
  - Endometrium
  - Fallopian tubes
  - Ovaries
  - Urethra
- Gonorrhea and chlamydia are most common causes
- Adolescent population accounts for 16–20% of all cases

Signs and Symptoms

- Severe abdominal pain
- Pain with ambulation
  - PID "shuffle"
    - Bent over at waist and clutching lower abdomen, causing a shuffling gait
- Purulent vaginal discharge
- Dysuria
- Fever

ED Treatment and Diagnostic Studies

- Airway, breathing and circulation (ABCs)
- Complete blood count (CBC), urine pregnancy test, UA, serologic testing to rule out syphilis
- Pelvic examination with appropriate cultures
- IV access as indicated
  - IV antibiotics
- Antipyretics and pain medication
- Ultrasound if indicated
- May be admitted to hospital or discharged home
- Instructions include use of condoms

URINARY TRACT INFECTION (UTI)

Upper Urinary Tract

- Ureters
- Renal pelvis
- Calyces
- Renal parenchyma

Lower Urinary Tract

- Bladder
- Urethra

UTI can involve upper and lower tracts

- More frequent in female patients
- *Escherichia coli* is the most common pathogen

Signs and Symptoms

- Burning
- Frequency
- Urgency
- Malodorous urine

- Child may pull at underwear or have increased frequency of accidents
  - "Pee-pee" dance

Systemic Symptoms

- Fever and chills
- Nausea and/or vomiting
- Malaise as exhibited by decreased activity or play

ED Treatment

- ABCs
- UA (clean-catch, catheterized, or suprapubic needle aspiration)
  - Culture urine as indicated by institution's policy
- IV access if indicated for IV antibiotic therapy or hydration
- Parental or caregiver instructions
  - No bubble baths
  - Change underwear frequently

HEMOLYTIC-UREMIC SYNDROME (HUS)

- An acute renal disease
- Causes
  - Intravascular coagulation
  - Renal failure
  - Hemolytic anemia
  - Thrombocytopenia
- Rare disease seen primarily in white children ages 6 mo–5 yr

Signs and Symptoms

- Linked prodromally with upper respiratory infection (URI) and GI symptoms
- Oliguria to anuria
- Nausea and vomiting

- Diarrhea
- Fever
- Hemolytic signs
  - Ecchymosis
  - Petechial rash
  - Hematuria
  - Jaundice
- Dehydration
- Hypertension to cardiac failure

ED Treatment

- ABCs
- CBC, chemistry, UA, cultures (blood and urine), coagulation studies
- IV access and fluid resuscitation as indicated
- Anticipate dialysis and blood or blood product administration
- Antibiotics as indicated

EPIDIDYMITIS

- Inflammation or an infection of the epididymis

Signs and Symptoms

- Swelling and enlargement of the epididymis
  - Causes scrotal swelling
- Usually unilateral, but could be bilateral
- Tenderness of the spermatic cord
- Fever
- Possible discharge from penis
- History of recent sexual activity

ED Treatment

- Emergency ultrasound of testicle to rule out torsion
- Elevation of testicles (relieves pain)
- Ice bag as tolerated
- Pain control

- Antibiotics and anti-inflammatory agents as indicated
- Protect privacy

TESTICULAR TORSION

- Twisting of the spermatic cord
- A true emergency that must be resolved within 6 hr to prevent testis death

Signs and Symptoms

- Severe pain and swelling of scrotum
- Positive Prehn's sign
  - Pain worsens with elevation of the testicle
- Tense scrotal mass
- Nausea and/or vomiting
- Fever

ED Treatment

- IV access
- Pain management
- Emergency ultrasound of testicles
- Manual manipulation or surgical intervention
  - Surgical preparation if manual manipulation is unsuccessful
- Must distinguish from epididymitis

HENOCH-SCHÖNLEIN PURPURA (HSP)

- Also known as anaphylactoid purpura or allergic purpura
- Associated with URI, allergic reactions, and/or drug sensitivities
- Seen in children ages 6 mo–16 yr
  - Male patients more often affected than females
- Is multisystem, but >50% of cases have renal involvement

Signs and Symptoms

- Symmetric maculopapular rash
  - Progresses to purpura and petechiae
- Joint swelling
  - Can be single, nonpainful joint
  - Can be several joints with pain
    - Knees
    - Ankles
- Abdominal pain
- Nausea and vomiting
- Heme-positive stools
- Hematuria

ED Treatment

- ABCs
- CBC, chemistry, UA
- Possible abdominal radiographs
- Pain management

Chapter 8
Hematologic/
Immunologic

SICKLE CELL DISEASE (SCD)

Description
- Group of genetic disorders characterized by
  - Production of sickle hemoglobin (HbS)
  - Chronic hemolytic anemia
  - Ischemic tissue injury
- Homozygous HbSS disease—sickle cell anemia
  - Most common form of SCD
  - Inherited autosomal recessive lifelong disease
  - Affects mostly African-Americans
    - 8% carry the sickle cell trait
    - Also seen in children of Middle Eastern and Mediterranean descent
  - ~25% of deaths related to SCD occur prior to 5th birthday
  - Diagnosis based on laboratory findings of sickled red blood cells (RBCs)
    - Hemoglobin electrophoresis
    - Elevated reticulocyte count—due to shortened lifespan of RBCs

Pathophysiology
- RBCs become sickled in shape, become inflexible, unable to flow through very small blood vessels during certain conditions
  - Low oxygen concentrations
  - Acidosis
  - Dehydration
- Sickled cells clump together, occluding vessels
- Oxygen will reverse sickling process, *but*

- Repeated sickling and unsickling causes cells to become irreversibly sickled
  - Further decreases lifespan of RBCs to ~12 days
- First signs and symptoms generally appear after 6 mo of age
  - Dactylitis
    - Unexplained swelling, apparent pain and decrease in use of hands and feet
    - Early vasoocclusive crisis
- Three types of crises
  - Vasoocclusive
  - Splenic sequestration
  - Aplastic
- Vasoocclusive
  - Microvascular occlusion
    - Tissue ischemia and necrosis, infarcts and organ damage
    - Organs affected
      - Lungs, spleen, brain—most severe
      - Liver, gut, extremities, back, penis
    - Triggered by stressors
      - Overexertion, infection, dehydration, acidosis, hypoxia, trauma

Signs and symptoms
- Irritability
- Pain—especially joints, all areas distal to occlusion
- Anorexia, vomiting
- Fever
- Decreased range of motion (ROM), warmth over affected area
- Leg ulcers
- Ocular hemorrhages

Emergency department (ED) treatment
- Pain control
  - Age-appropriate play, imagery, distraction
  - Oral or IV analgesia
    - IV narcotics

- Morphine is the drug of choice: 0.1–0.2 mg/kg (maximum = 10 mg)
- Continuous infusion of IV morphine
  - Use of patient-controlled analgesia pump
- Evaluation of pain control measures
  - Every 1–2 hr
  - Age-appropriate pain assessment tool (see Section I, Reference 20. Wong-Baker Faces Pain Rating Scale)
- Hydration—dependent on severity of symptoms
  - Oral
  - IV fluids at one and a half to two times maintenance (see Table 5–4)
    - Monitor for signs and symptoms of fluid overload
- Antibiotics specific to infection
- Warm compresses to affected areas
- Rest, comfort measures
- Oxygen—does *not* reverse sickling process
  - Maintain $SpO_2 \geq 95\%$
  - Long-term oxygen therapy may decrease bone marrow activity and actually worsen the anemia

SELECTED VASOOCCLUSIVE CRISES IN SCD

Acute chest syndrome

- May be life threatening accompanied by respiratory distress
- May be confused with pneumonia
  - Pulmonary infiltrates not uncommon
  - May recur
  - Usually in children >12 yr old
  - Usual trigger is infection

Signs and symptoms
- As previously cited for vasoocclusive crisis
- Chest pain

- Dyspnea, cough
- Leukocytosis
- Pleural rub, pleural effusion

ED treatment
- As previously cited for vasoocclusive crisis
- Oxygen
- Nebulized respiratory treatments
- Ongoing respiratory and cardiac assessments
- Position for comfort
- Encourage deep breathing, although the child may resist due to pain
  - Ensure adequate pain control
- RBC transfusions as needed to increase oxygen-carrying capacity of the blood
- Prepare for diagnostic procedures
  - Chest x-ray
  - Ventilation/perfusion scan
  - Electrocardiogram, laboratory draws, arterial blood gases
- Prepare for admission and/or transfer

Stroke

- Thrombolytic or hemorrhagic
- May recur

Signs and symptoms
- As previously cited for vasoocclusive crisis
- Alteration in level of consciousness, usual behavior
- Severe headache, visual alterations
- Slurred speech
- Ataxia, seizures
- Paresthesias, paralysis
- Nuchal rigidity
- Xanthochromic spinal fluid

ED treatment
- As previously cited for vasoocclusive crisis
- Long-term transfusion therapy

- 90% effective in preventing recurrent strokes
- Continued indefinitely
- May present to ED with signs of iron toxicity/ iron overload from long-term transfusion therapy
  - Iron deposits on organs with resultant
    - Cardiomyopathy
    - Cirrhosis
    - Insulin-dependent diabetes mellitus
    - Hypothyroidism
    - Hypoparathyroidism
    - Delayed growth and development
  - May require chelation therapy with deferoxamine (Desferal)

Splenic sequestration crisis

- Large portion of peripheral blood pools in spleen
  - Splenic enlargement
  - Severe anemia
  - Hypovolemic shock—life-threatening
- Most common 6 mo–4 yr old (before splenic autoinfarction)
- Trigger may be viral illness or infection
- May recur

Signs and symptoms
- Pallor
- Irritability
- May exhibit signs of profound shock
- Tachycardia
- Priapism
- Splenomegaly
- Low hemoglobin level

ED treatment
- Initiate measures to stabilize airway, breathing, and circulation (ABCs)
- IV fluids: Initial bolus, 2 mL/kg of isotonic solution

- Frequent assessments for circulatory over-load
- RBC transfusions to restore circulating blood volume
  - 5–10 mL/kg over 3–4 hr if stable
- Supplemental oxygen, maintain $SpO_2 \geq 95\%$
- Ongoing assessments of ABCs, level of consciousness (LOC)
- Prepare for admission
  - Eventual splenectomy may be necessary

Aplastic crisis

- Associated with infection by human parvovirus
- Rapid destruction of RBCs
- Impaired RBC production in bone marrow
  - Profound anemia
  - High-output congestive heart failure (CHF)

Signs and symptoms
- Pallor, scleral icterus
- Lethargy, fatigue, weakness
- Headache
- Fainting
- Anorexia
- Tachycardia
- Recent respiratory infection
- Decreased reticulocyte count

ED treatment
- IV fluids
- Blood transfusions
- Frequent assessments for fluid overload
- Prepare for admission

Prevention/family education
- Focus of therapy
  - Prevention of infection
  - Treat anemia
  - Prevent vasoocclusive episodes
- Daily penicillin
- *Haemophilus influenzae* vaccine

- Pneumococcal vaccine
- Hepatitis B vaccine
- Signs and symptoms of an infection
- How to take the child's temperature at home
- Encourage fluid intake: one and a half to two times daily requirement
- Stress management
- Physical, emotional, and cold stress
- Ensure adequate rest
- Importance of regular physician/clinic visits and follow-up care
  - Development of a self-management plan to treat vasoocclusive crisis at home
  - Specific written directions regarding when to seek help in the ED
- Participation in sports, gym classes—prevent strenuous exertion, which may result in hypoxia
- Psychosocial and emotional support for child and parents
- Referrals to genetic counseling, support groups
  - American Sickle Cell Anemia Association
    10300 Carnegie Avenue
    Cleveland, OH 44106
    (216) 229-8600

HEMOPHILIA

- Hereditary bleeding disorder
- Chronic, no cure
- Specific clotting factors are missing or defective
  - Factor VIII—antihemophiliac factor (classic hemophilia)
  - Factor IX—plasma thromboplastin component (Christmas disease)
- Bleeding times prolonged
  - Increased risk for hemarthrosis, hemorrhage
- Majority of children diagnosed as neonates
  - Prolonged umbilical cord or circumcision bleeding, severe cephalohematoma

- Severity classifications
  - Mild—usually only noted after severe trauma or surgery
  - Moderate—associated with bleeding after minor trauma
  - Severe—spontaneous bleeding episodes
- Specific hemophilia history to obtain in ED
  - Baseline factor level
  - Time and dose of last factor infusion
  - Inhibitor history
  - Acetylsalicylic acid (ASA) or nonsteroidal anti-inflammatory drug use
  - Allergy to concentrates

Bleeding episodes in hemophilia

- Major sites of serious bleeding
  - Spinal cord
  - Throat
  - Intraabdominal
  - Ocular
  - Limb compartments
- Characterized by bleeding into an enclosed space
- Compression of vital tissue
- Potential loss of life, limb, function

Hemarthrosis—bleeding into joint spaces, and muscle bleeding

- May result in permanent damage
- Degenerative changes, decrease in ROM
- Nerve compression and muscle fibrosis
- Signs and symptoms
  - Joint or muscle pain
  - Decreased ROM, movement
  - Swelling, unequal limb girth
  - Bruising, warmth over area
    Evidence of bruising or surface trauma is *not* necessary to confirm bleeding into joint or muscle
  - Areas most commonly affected

- Knee, elbow, ankle, shoulder, hip
- Forearm, flexor, gastrocnemius, iliopsoas

ED treatment
- Ascertain if child is being followed in a hemophiliac treatment center
  - If yes, parent often will have individualized written emergency treatment plan
- Administration of factor VIII or IX
  - Dose dependent on factor deficiency, patient's weight, and amount of bleeding (Table 8–1)
- Pain control
  - Distraction, imagery, age-appropriate play
  - Avoid IM injections
  - Narcotic analgesics, avoid ASA
    - Oral or IV established for administration of factor
- Cold packs to affected area
- Immobilization and elevation of affected area
  - Sling and splint application, as appropriate
- Pad side rails, safety measures to prevent bleeding episodes
- Ongoing assessments
  - Pain relief—use age-appropriate pain assessment tool (see Section I, Reference 20. Wong-Baker Faces Pain Rating Scale)
  - Vital signs
  - LOC
  - Signs and symptoms of continued bleeding
  - Distal neurovascular status
  - Signs and symptoms of compartment syndrome (see Chapter 11, Orthopedic)
- Minimize invasive procedures
  - Use IV catheter with smallest diameter to infuse factor
  - Obtain laboratory specimens at time of IV placement
  - Apply pressure after all venipunctures
  - Do not take rectal temperatures
  - Arthrocentesis

Table 8–1. Recommended Dosages of Factor VIII and Factor IX*

Type of Bleeding	Initial Dose (Factor IX U/kg Source of Factor IX)	Repeated Dose (Factor IX U/kg Source of Factor IX)	Initial Dose (U/kg) Factor VIII	Repeated Dose (U/kg) Factor VIII
Acute hemarthrosis	Mild: 15 mL/kg FFP Severe: 20–30 FIXCC	Severe: 20–25 FIXCC in 24 hr	20	20 in 12 or 24 hr
Intramuscular	Mild: 15 mL/kg FFP Severe: 20–30 FIXCC	Mild: 10–15 mL/kg FFP every 24 hr Severe: 20–30 FIXCC every 24 hr	20–30	20 every 12 hr
Subcutaneous	10 mL/kg FFP 10 FIXCC	Rarely needed	10	Rarely needed
Life threatening; CNS, major trauma, bleeding with potential airway obstruction, retroperitoneal, GI, surgery	50 FIXCC	20–25 FIXCC every 24 hr	50	25–30 every 8–12 hr
Gross hematuria	20 FIXCC	20 FIXCC every 24 hr	20	20 every 12 hr
Tongue and mouth	30–40 FIXCC	May be necessary Also consider Amicar	20	Often necessary Also consider beginning Amicar 100 mg/kg/dose

*Consider administration of factor before spinal tap, IM injections, laceration repair, and with head injuries without evidence of CNS bleeding.
FFP = fresh frozen plasma; FIXCC = factor IX complex concentrate.
Modified from Barkin P, Rosen P: Emergency Pediatrics, 4th ed. St. Louis, Mosby–Year Book, 1994.

- May be necessary if distal neurovascular status is compromised
- Administer factor before joint aspiration
- Risk of rebleeding
- Disposition
  - Most children are discharged to home
    - Maintain cold packs, immobilization
    - Observe at home for signs of continued bleeding or rebleeding
    - Consider leaving IV catheter in place for parents to administer repeat dose(s) of factor at home
      - Usually given 12–24 hr after first dose, if necessary
      - Evaluate risks and benefits of discharging with saline lock in place
        - Parental readiness
        - Parental supervision
        - Follow up with primary physician
          - Catheter removal
  - Prepare for admission if associated with compartment syndrome or neurovascular compromise

Prevention/family education
- Avoid medications that may prolong bleeding times
  - ASA, ibuprofen, indomethacin, phenylbutazone, guaifenesin
- Psychosocial and emotional support for child and family
  - Referrals, resources
    - National Hemophilia Foundation
      The Sotto Building
      110 Greene Street, Suite 406
      New York, NY 10012
      (212) 219-8180
      www.infonhf.org

Central nervous system (CNS)—
Intracranial or spinal cord
- Spontaneous or due to trauma

- High morbidity and mortality
- Subdural, epidural, subarachnoid, intraventricular, intracerebral
- Signs and symptoms—determined by site of bleeding
  - Nausea and vomiting
  - Irritability
  - Sustained headache (>4 hr)
  - Nuchal rigidity
  - Change in behavior, LOC
  - Slurred speech
  - Ataxia
  - Visual disturbances
  - Muscle weakness, paralysis
  - Paresthesias
  - Seizures
- Diagnostic studies
  - Computed tomography (CT)
  - Magnetic resonance imaging (MRI)

ED treatment
- As for hemarthrosis, and
- ABCs
- IV access with laboratory specimens drawn at same time
- Primary intervention is always factor replacement
  - Do not wait for laboratory results
- Ongoing assessments
  - ABCs
  - LOC
  - Vital signs
  - Complete assessment
    - Other areas with hematomas, ecchymosis, other evidence of bleeding, trauma
  - Elevate head of bed 30°
  - Assess for IV fluid overload

Pharyngeal bleeds—
Densely vascular area

- Nasopharynx—minor threat unless associated with large blood volume loss

- Oropharynx or laryngopharynx—may be acute respiratory emergency

ED treatment
- As for hemarthrosis, and
- Ensure airway patency
- ABCs
- IV access with laboratory specimens drawn at same time¨
- Primary intervention is always factor replacement
- Apply pressure to nose for 15 min
- Position sitting upright, may lean forward
- Cauterization or nasal packing as indicated
- Assess ability to swallow saliva
- Lateral neck radiographs to assess for presence of mass
- Consider ear, nose, and throat (ENT) consultation
- Ongoing assessments of airway patency and respiratory status
- Disposition
  - May be able to discharge to home with clear instructions
    - Observe at home and return to ED immediately if
      - Difficulty breathing
      - Neck swelling
      - Inability to swallow
      - Change in voice
      - Choking
      - Change in color

Prevention/family education
- Avoid straws, hot fluids
- No running or other activities while anything is in mouth (e.g., sucker)

Abdominal bleeds

- Abdominal pain may be associated with
  - GI tract hematomas

- Pseudotumors
- Iliopsoas or retroperitoneal bleeding
- Abdomen may sequester significant amounts of blood with little external evidence of bleeding

Signs and symptoms
- Abdominal pain
  - May be associated with hip or groin pain
  - May be accompanied by inability to bear weight on one leg
- Dizziness, syncope
- Shortness of breath
- Nausea, vomiting
- Rectal bleeding, hematemesis
- Tachycardia, increased respiratory rate
- Cool, moist skin

ED treatment
- As for hemarthrosis, and
- ABCs
- IV access with laboratory specimens drawn at same time
- Primary intervention is always factor replacement
- Focused history to include
  - Past surgeries, trauma, previous abdominal bleeding
- Focused assessment and ongoing assessments
  - ABCs
  - Level of consciousness
  - Vital signs
  - Skin color, temperature, moisture
  - Capillary refill
  - Abdominal swelling, ecchymosis, masses, pulsations, contours
  - Presence of bowel sounds in all quadrants
  - *Gentle* palpation for tenderness, hematoma
  - ROM of hips
  - Presence of occult blood in stool, presence of microscopic hematuria

Intraocular bleeding

- Most commonly associated with trauma, may be spontaneous

Signs and symptoms
- Focused history to include
  - Prior bleeding episodes or eye complications
- Pain
- Change in visual acuity
- Diplopia
- Blurred or lost vision
- Photophobia
- Itching, tearing, discharge

ED treatment
- Primary intervention is always factor replacement
- Rest eye
  - Patch
- Cold compresses
- Darkened room
- Ophthalmology consult

Prevention/family education
- Wear protective eyewear during any activity with flying objects (e.g., baseball, tennis)
- Do not run while carrying objects

HIV/AIDS

Description
- By the year 2000, an estimated 10 million children will be infected with HIV (40 million people worldwide)
- 1995—more than 6000 children in the United States were reported to have AIDS
- Vertical (mother to child) transmission is most common (80% of cases)
  - In utero, intrapartum, or postnatally by breast-feeding (up to 15%)
  - Treatment of infected pregnant women and

newborns after birth with zidovudine (ZDT) has proven to reduce transmission rate

- Infection via blood products continues in underdeveloped countries
- Sexual abuse by HIV-positive perpetrator
- Adolescents and older children
  - Transmission from heterosexual and homosexual activities
  - Use of shared injection equipment
- Virus predominantly affects the T4 lymphocyte (CD4 + - T helper cells)
  - Also affects macrophages, neuronal and glial cells in CNS
- Infected neonates appear normal at birth
  - May be small for gestational age or premature
- Presentation of HIV infection varies; in general, more rapidly progressive in children than in adults
  - "Rapid progressors"—children who develop AIDS and die within the 1st year of life
  - "Slow progressors"—children in whom the disease progresses more slowly; many live to their teenage years

Diagnosis
- 95% of infected children are diagnosed by age 6 mo
- Children born to HIV-infected mothers will have maternal HIV antibody present at birth and detectable until 10–18 mo
- Enzyme-linked immunosorbent assay (ELISA) test may show false-positive results until after maternal antibodies are lost
  - Two negative ELISA tests will confirm the infant is not infected
  - Child older than 18 mo with a positive ELISA is HIV infected
- Polymerase chain reaction (PCR) test detects the HIV genome
  - As infection may occur late in pregnancy or

at time of delivery; a negative result in the first 2–3 mo of life does not exclude infection
- Viral cultures for HIV—the "gold standard" for diagnosis in infants
- Diagnosis of HIV infection may be made in children <18 mo with presence of HIV in two separate blood samples drawn at different times
- Other laboratory indicators of infection
  - High immunoglobulin levels
  - Reversed CD4+/CD8+ T-lymphocyte ratio
  - Low CD4+ levels for age

Signs and symptoms—children younger than 13 yr
- Classifications based on Center for Disease Control symptom classification
- Mild
  - Lymphadenopathy
  - Hepatomegaly
  - Splenomegaly
  - Dermatitis
  - Parotitis
  - Recurrent or persistent upper respiratory tract infection, sinusitis, or otitis media
- Moderate
  - Anemia
  - Neutropenia
  - Diarrhea
  - Persistent fever of unknown origin
  - Herpes stomatitis
  - Oral candidiasis
  - Bacterial meningitis, pneumonia, sepsis
  - Cardiomyopathy
  - Complicated varicella
  - Hepatitis
  - Nephropathy
  - Herpes zoster
  - Lymphocytic interstitial pneumonia (LIP)
    - Rare in adults
    - Initially asymptomatic

- Diagnosed by persistent abnormal chest x-ray, often in 2nd year of life
- Severe (most common)
  - Multiple or recurrent bacterial infections
    - Especially *Streptococcus pneumoniae, H. influenzae, Salmonella*
    - Pneumonia is most common infection
  - *Pneumocystic carinii* pneumonia (PCP)
    - Most common opportunistic infection
    - Most frequent between 3–6 mo of age
    - High mortality
  - Cytomegalovirus (CMV)
  - Encephalophathy
    - Motor developmental delays
    - Language delays
    - Behavioral abnormalities and memory loss in older children
  - Wasting syndrome
    - Secondary to infections, poor intake or enteropathy
- Immune category—see Table 8–2
  - Most common cause of death in infected children is opportunistic bacterial or viral infections leading to respiratory failure
    - Prophylaxis against opportunistic infections (especially PCP)
      - Begin at 4–6 wk of age and continue until 1 year
    - Children with PCP, CMV, encephalopathy, and lymphoma have higher mortality than those with LIP and bacterial infections

ED treatment
- Focused on aggressive treatment of the HIV-related infection that prompted the ED visit
- Nonjudgmental approach to care of the child and family
- Ensure confidentiality
- Psychosocial and emotional support for child and family
  - Frequently the HIV-infected mother must deal with her child's death before she exhib-

Table 8–2. Immune Category—Based on Age and CD4 Count

Immune Category	CD4+ Count 0–11 mo	CD4+ Count 1–5 yr	CD4+ Count 6–12 yr
No evidence of suppression	>1500	>1000	>500
Moderate suppression	750–1499	500–999	200–499
Severe suppression	<750	<500	<200

Modified from Centers for Disease Control: 1994 revised classification system for human immunodeficiency virus infection in children less than 13 years of age. Morb Mortal Wkly Rep 43:1–10, 1994.

its serious HIV-related health problems herself
- Allow expressions of guilt, anger, denial, anticipatory grieving
- Referrals and resources
  - Local support groups, community agencies
  - AIDS hotline: (800) 342-2437
  - National Pediatric HIV Resource Center
    15 South 9th Street
    Newark, NJ 07107
    (201) 268-8251; (800) 362-0071
- Antiretroviral agents for HIV infection
  - Inhibit HIV replication
  - ZDT
    - Orally, or IV if child is to receive nothing PO
  - Didanosine
- Protease inhibitors are becoming more common in children

NEUTROPENIA

- Neutropenia is an absolute neutrophil count (ANC) of $<1500/mm^3$
  ANC = (% neutrophils + % bands) $\times$ white blood cell count
- Hereditary or acquired
  - Secondary to specific infections, toxins, drugs
    - Immunosuppressant drug therapy
      - Cancer treatments, antirejection therapy following transplantation
- Places child at high risk for serious, often life-threatening infection
- Child with fever and neutropenia is triaged as emergent
  - Bacteria multiply rapidly
  - Overwhelming sepsis occurs very quickly
  - Severity of neutropenia
    - Little or no risk of infection: ANC >1000
    - Moderate risk of infection: ANC 500–1000
    - Significant risk of infection: ANC <500
    - Profound risk of infection: ANC <300

- Diagnostic studies
  - Laboratory specimens
    - Complete blood count with differential
    - Chemistries
    - Platelet count
    - Prothrombin time/partial thromboplastin time (PT/PTT)
    - Type and cross-match
    - Urinalysis
  - Cultures
    - Blood via venipuncture
    - Blood taken from implanted port or each lumen of central line (if applicable)
    - Urine
    - Wound (if applicable)
  - Chest x-ray

ED treatment
- Place child in as private an area as is available
  - Avoid contact with potentially infectious persons, especially other patients with varicella
- ABCs
- Vascular access with laboratory specimens
- Vital signs
- Continuous monitoring of noninvasive blood pressure, heart rate, pulse oximetry
- Intake and output
- Ongoing assessment
  - Level of consciousness
  - Skin color, temperature, moisture
  - Capillary refill
  - Temperature
  - Fluid status
  - Development of rash
- Maintain pulse oximetry >95%
- No unnecessary invasive procedures
  - No rectal temperatures or suppositories
  - Minimize venipunctures
- Administer antipyretics
- Administer antibiotics

Selected Bibliography

Ashwill JW, Droske SC: Nursing Care of Children: Principles and Practice. Philadelphia, W.B. Saunders, 1997.

Barkin R, Rosen P: Emergency Pediatrics: A Guide to Ambulatory Care, 4th ed. St. Louis, Mosby–Year Book, 1994.

Betz CL, Sowden LA: Mosby's Pediatric Nursing Reference, 3rd ed. St. Louis, Mosby–Year Book, 1996.

Davies E, Elliman D, Hart C, et al.: Manual of Childhood Infections. Philadelphia, W. B. Saunders, 1996.

Soud TE, Rogers JS: Manual of Pediatric Emergency Nursing. Philadelphia, Mosby–Year Book, 1998.

Chapter 9
Maltreatment

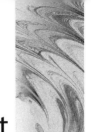

- Major types
  - Physical
  - Sexual
  - Emotional
  - Neglect
- More than 1000 children die annually as a result of maltreatment
- Maltreatment crosses all racial, ethnic, socio-economic, religious, and geographic groups
- There is no "formula" to predict maltreatment
- Certain characteristics are more frequently observed in abused or neglected children (Table 9–1)
- Nurses are mandated by law to report suspected child maltreatment in the United States

Table 9–1. Characteristics Associated With Child Maltreatment

Child

Prematurity
Developmental delays
Congenital anomalies, physical disability
Chronic illness
Perception of being a "difficult" child

Caregiver

Alcohol or drug abuse
Lack of parenting experience, poor parenting models
Limited resources—financial, emotional
History of maltreatment as a child
Social isolation
Unrealistic expectations of child
Situational stress—acute or chronic

- Specific child welfare agencies vary from state to state

PHYSICAL ABUSE— NONACCIDENTAL PHYSICAL INJURY OR TRAUMA

- Most common injuries
  - Bruises, burns, fractures, head trauma, eye injury

Signs and Symptoms

- Bruising
  - On unusual areas of body
  - Face, neck, chest, abdomen, back, flank, thighs
  - In various stages of healing
  - Bruising patterns of identifiable objects
    - Looped cords, belt buckles, hand, coat hanger, sticks
- Human bite marks
- Burns
  - Immersion burns—circumferential or "stocking" burns on extremities
  - Cigarette burns
  - Pattern burns
    - Cigarette lighter, curling iron, steam clothes iron, radiator
  - Dunking burns—usually of buttocks and genitalia
    - Especially if child is of toilet training age
  - Burns on soles of feet, palms of hands
  - Rope burns on wrists or ankles
- Squeeze, pinch, or suck marks
- Head injuries
  - Most common type of nonaccidental trauma in infants
  - Shaken impact syndrome
    - Associated with cerebral edema and retinal hemorrhages

- Bilateral fractures or any fractures in an infant
- Subdural and subarachnoid bleeding common
- Traction alopecia from pulling child's hair
- Fractures and dislocations
  - Facial fractures
  - Spiral fractures from twisting the child's extremity, transverse fractures
  - Multiple fractures, both old and new
  - Fractures of ribs, scapula, sternum
- Other
  - Hyphema, retinal detachment
  - Persistent vomiting, abdominal pain
  - Hematuria

Diagnostic Studies

- Obtain complete history
- Physical examination of fully undressed child
- Specific x-rays of suspected injuries
- Long bone radiographic survey, "skeletal survey"
  - Fractures in various stages of healing are consistent with abuse
- Coagulation studies
  - Rule out blood dyscrasias, leukemia, hemophilia
  - Complete blood count with platelet count
  - Prothrombin time/partial thromboplastin time (PT/PTT)
  - Urinalysis

Emergency Department (ED) Treatment

- Assessment and stabilization of specific injuries
- Identification of maltreatment
- Mandated report to proper agency
- Evidence collection

- Photographs taken in ED as part of medical record and/or by law enforcement agency
- Forensic photographs include a rule and complete patient data
- Documentation in medical record
  - Size, shape, location, and description of all obvious injuries
  - Document exact child and caregiver statements verbatim, using quotations
  - Ensure chain of evidence according to local policy for any evidence collected
- Communicate suspicions to caregivers
  - Communication is nonjudgmental and caring
  - Allow caregiver to ask questions
  - Explain what will happen next
- Ensure confidentiality
- Disposition
  - Consult with multidisciplinary team members
    - Social worker, child life specialist, law enforcement agency, child protection service
  - Admission or discharge is based on
    - Child's medical condition/injuries
    - Safety of home environment, prevention of further abuse
      - Protective custody may be an option, dependent on specific state laws

SEXUAL ABUSE

- The use or coercion of any child to engage in sexually explicit conduct
- Perpetrator is known to the child in 80% of cases
- Acute or chronic
- Interviewing
  - Techniques and choice of interviewer vary among jurisdictions and institutions
  - In general, an experienced interviewer should elicit specific history related to sexual abuse

- Avoid multiple interviews
- Never interview the child in front of possible perpetrator
- Use a quiet, private room; establish trust and rapport
- Use child's own terminology for body parts and actions
- Use age-appropriate tools (e.g., anatomically correct dolls, drawings)

Signs and Symptoms

- Trauma to genitalia, anus, mouth or throat
  - Bruises, bleeding, lacerations
- Soiled, stained, bloody underwear
- Dysuria, frequent urinary tract infections
- Discomfort or itching in genital area
- Sexually transmitted disease (STD) in child <12 yr (usually not yet sexually active)
  - Vaginal discharge, penile discharge
- Pregnancy in young adolescent
- Behavioral characteristics
  - Excessive masturbation; preoccupation with sexual matters
  - Poor relationships with peers
  - Sleep disorders, nightmares
  - Poor school performance
  - Regressive behaviors
  - Depression; suicidal ideation, attempts
  - Substance abuse
  - Running away from home

Diagnostic Studies

- Same as Previously Cited for Physical Abuse
- Genital examination
  - Girls examined in frog-leg position
- Pelvic examination/colposcopy
  - Never force or hold a child down for the examination

- Consider examination at another time in another setting
- Consider examination under anesthesia
- Anal examination
  - Lateral decubitus position
- Culture for STDs
- Evaluate for HIV exposure/infection
- Collection of fluid to examine for the presence of sperm
- Pregnancy test

ED Treatment

- Same as Previously Cited for Physical Abuse
- Treatment for STDs as indicated
- Pregnancy prophylaxis/referral if pregnant
- Referral to a center for comprehensive evaluation of sexually abused child
- Disposition—same as previously cited for physical abuse

EMOTIONAL ABUSE

- Often most difficult type of abuse to prove
- May involve unusual punishment
- Aggressive or berating remarks by the caregiver to the child
- Results in low self-esteem

Signs and Symptoms

- Failure to thrive
- Bed wetting
- Sleep disorders
- Behavioral characteristics
  - Self-stimulatory behaviors—rocking, sucking
  - Withdrawal
  - Antisocial behaviors
  - Suicide ideation, attempts

NEGLECT

- Intentional or unintentional lack of provision of basic needs of child
- Types of neglect
  - Medical
  - Physical
  - Emotional
  - Educational
  - Mental health
  - 45% of all abuse cases involve neglect

Signs and Symptoms

- Failure to thrive without identifiable medical cause
- Malnutrition
- Developmental delays
- Poor hygiene
  - Assess child's dentition
  - Feces and dirt in skin folds
  - Severe diaper rash with ammonia burns
- Lack of or inadequate health care
- Injuries due to lack of supervision
- Multiple dog or cat bites and scratches
- Inappropriate dress for weather
- Behavioral characteristics
  - Inactivity
  - Older children: stealing, absenteeism from school, substance abuse

Selected Bibliography

Betz CL, Sowden LA: Mosby's Pediatric Nursing Reference, 3rd ed. St. Louis, Mosby–Year Book, 1996.

Haley K, Baker P (eds): Instructor Manual: Emergency Nursing Pediatric Course. Chicago, Emergency Nurses Association, 1993.

Newberry L: Sheehy's Emergency Nursing: Principles and Practice, 4th ed. St. Louis, Mosby–Year Book, 1998.

Soud TE, Rogers JS: Manual of Pediatric Emergency Nursing. St. Louis, Mosby–Year Book, 1998.

Wong D: Whaley and Wong's Nursing Care of Infants and Children, 5th ed. St. Louis, Mosby–Year Book, 1995.

Chapter 10
Neurologic

SEIZURES

- Seizure: transient abnormal, excessive discharge of electrical neuronal activity
  - Extent of seizure dependent on location and amount of abnormal cerebral electrical discharge with alterations in motor, sensory, autonomic function, and/or consciousness
  - Causes
    - Cerebral
    - Encephalopathy
      - Hemorrhage
      - Infection
      - Trauma
      - Developmental defects
    - Biochemical
      - Metabolic disorders
      - Toxins
    - Posttraumatic
    - Idiopathic
      - No identifiable cause can be found

Definitions
- Prolonged seizure: lasting >15 min
- Status epilepticus: repetitive tonic-clonic seizures without regaining consciousness between, or single seizure lasting >30 min
  - At risk for airway obstruction, respiratory depression, hypoxia, hypotension, acidosis, increased intracranial pressure, hypoglycemia and hyperthermia
  - A medical emergency
- Epilepsy: chronic, recurrent seizure activity

- Partial (focal, local) seizures: abnormal discharges in one area or hemisphere of the brain
  - Simple partial seizures: no alteration of consciousness
  - Complex partial seizures: impairment of consciousness
    - May demonstrate automatisms (e.g., lip smacking, chewing, repetitive picking) or not (e.g., staring)
- Generalized (petit mal, grand mal) seizures involve all or majority of cerebral cortex
  - Convulsive
    - Myoclonic: sudden jerking of a muscle or muscle group, lasting <5 sec; momentary loss of consciousness
    - Tonic-clonic: loss of consciousness, stiffening of limb muscles; may include loss of bowel or bladder control, followed by clonic movements of extremities; may include hypoxia, apnea, and cyanosis; postictal phase includes confusion and often sleep
  - Nonconvulsive
    - Absence seizures: impaired awareness and responsiveness, staring lasting less than 15 sec
    - Atonic seizures: sudden loss of tone; may fall to the ground
- Neonatal seizures
  - Occur within the 1st mo of life
  - May be difficult to diagnose when characterized by frequent, subtle movements of lips, eyes, or extremities
  - Causes: perinatal hypoxia, birth trauma, metabolic disorders, infection, structural abnormalities, drug withdrawal
- Infantile spasms
  - Occur 3 mo–2 yr of age
  - Cryptogenic: No apparent cause
  - Symptomatic: Etiology related to fetal development, delivery, postnatal or maternal factors

- Characterized by brief spasms of neck, trunk, and extremities, which may occur in clusters
- >80% of infants are mentally retarded

Diagnostic Data (Influenced by History and Clinical Presentation)

- Febrile child (see following section on febrile seizures)
- Trauma (see following section on head injury)
- Intoxication: Include serum and urine drug screens
- Abnormalities in growth and development (see following section on shunt malfunction)
- All children with seizures should have initial bedside glucose determination
- Other laboratory tests include complete blood count (CBC) with differential and electrolytes
- Consider computed tomography (CT) scan, possibly magnetic resonance imaging (MRI), especially with continued abnormal neurologic findings
- Electroencephalogram (EEG) is of little or no value in the emergency department (ED)
- If known seizure disorder and on antiepileptics: serum drug levels
  - Selected antiepileptic drugs include
    - Carbamazepine (Tegretol)
    - Clonazepam (Klonopin)
    - Ethosuximide (Zarontin)
    - Gabapentin (Neurontin)
    - Lamotrigine (Lamictal)
    - Mephobarbital (Mebaral)
    - Phenobarbital (Barbita)
    - Phenytoin (Dilantin)
    - Primidone (Mysoline)
    - Valproic acid (Depakene)
- Febrile seizures
  - Generalized tonic-clonic seizures associated with a fever, usually in children 5 mo–5 yr

- Last <15 min and generally followed by a postictal period
- When fully awake, a normal level of consciousness is evident
- The majority of pediatric seizures treated in the ED
- Usually <6 yr
- 30% risk of a subsequent febrile seizure
- Thought to be precipitated by the amount and rapidity of rise in body temperature
- Parental history of preceding illness with fever is typical
- 70–90% are associated with otitis media, pharyngitis, adenitis, or pneumonitis
- Seizures are self-limited
- Always consider meningitis or a serious bacterial infection in the febrile child with seizures
  - Assess for
    - Meningeal irritation
    - Petechiae
    - Decreased level of consciousness
- Diagnostic data for first-time suspected febrile seizure may include
  - Lumbar puncture
  - Test cerebrospinal fluid (CSF) for: cell count, Gram stain, culture, protein and glucose
- Serum glucose, electrolytes, blood urea nitrogen
- CBC with differential

ED treatment
- Airway, breathing, and circulation (ABCs)
  - Actively seizing child
    - Position on side if not contraindicated
    - Protect the child from injury
    - Suction as needed; maintain patency of airway
    - Administer oxygen, 100% by mask

- Bag and mask ventilate if ventilation is inadequate
- If seizure does not stop quickly, initiate IV access to administer anticonvulsants (Table 10–1)
- IM and rectal routes of drug administration are slow and unreliable
- When the drugs cited here do not halt seizure activity, prepare for intubation and controlled ventilation
- Pentobarbital (barbiturate coma)
  - Usually initiated after admission to intensive care unit (ICU) if necessary
  - Loading dose: 5 mg/kg IV slowly every 5 minutes while observing EEG, to a maximum of 20 mg/kg
- Institute seizure precautions if not actively seizing on arrival
  - Padded side rails or crib pads
  - Suction at bedside
  - Airway equipment at bedside
  - Appropriate size bag, valve, mask device at bedside
  - Oxygen at bedside
- Documentation
  - Clear description of seizure activity
    - Loss of consciousness
    - Length of seizure
    - Areas of body involved
    - Loss of bowel or bladder control in age-appropriate child
    - Postictal state
  - Vital signs and neurologic assessment with descriptions of deficits
  - Past history of seizures
  - Family history of febrile seizures
  - General condition prior to seizure
  - Medications
  - Possible exposures
  - Possible ingestion
  - Recent trauma, head injury

Table 10–1. Selected Anticonvulsants for the Actively Seizing Child

Drug	Dose	Onset	Duration	Comments
Lorazepam	0.05–0.1 mg/kg (maximum, 4 mg)	2–8 min	3–24 hr	Initial drug of choice May repeat in 10 min if no response Rectal: 0.01 mg/kg Assess for respiratory depression, hypotension, and sedation
Diazepam	0.1–0.3 mg/kg (maximum, 10 mg)	1–2 min	20–30 min	Assess for respiratory depression, hypotension, and sedation
Midazolam	0.1–0.3 mg/kg (maximum, 5–10 mg)	1–5 min	<2 hr	Assess for respiratory depression, hypotension, and sedation
Phenytoin	20 mg/kg slowly (1 mg/kg/min)	15–30 min	>24 hr	Less sedating; assess for hypotension and conduction defects; if given too rapidly, bradycardia and hypotension may occur
Phenobarbital	20 mg/kg	20–30 min	>24 hr	Synergistic with benzodiazepines; assess for sedation and respiratory depression

Modified from Singh N: Manual of Pediatric Critical Care. Philadelphia, W.B. Saunders, 1997.

- Congenital or other neurologic disorders
- Encourage family members to remain with the child

Disposition
- Anticipate discharge to home
  - Child with chronic seizure disorder
    - Subtherapeutic antiepileptic medications
      - Adjustment of dosage may be necessary with scheduled follow-up
      - Observation in ED prior to discharge
  - Child with febrile seizure
    - Non–life-threatening infection
    - Parental understanding of antibiotic and antipyretic administration, scheduled follow-up
- Anticipate admission to hospital or transfer to pediatric facility
  - First seizure, unknown cause
  - Status epilepticus
  - Complicating factors
    - Intoxication
    - Head injury
    - Cerebral pathology
    - Severe infection (e.g., meningitis, sepsis)
    - Metabolic disorders (e.g., hyponatremia)
- Prevention
  - Parental education
    - Administration of antipyretics for febrile seizures
    - Prevention of injury to child during seizure
      - Do not force anything into mouth
      - Prevention of aspiration
    - Importance of regular medical visits to adjust anticonvulsants as child grows
    - Activities that may need restrictions (e.g., swimming, driving, climbing)
    - Potential triggers
      - Loud noises, flashing or flickering lights
      - Drug or alcohol consumption
      - Illness, stress

- Referral to
National Epilepsy Foundation of America
4351 Garden City Drive
Landover, MD 20785
800-EFA-1000
Fax: (301) 577-4941

HYDROCEPHALUS AND VENTRICULOPERITONEAL (VP) SHUNT EMERGENCIES

Hydrocephalus

- Shunting of CSF from the ventricles will reduce accumulation and reduce potential irreversible brain damage
  - Insertion of a VP shunt is most common
    - Proximal end is inserted into lateral ventricle and attached to a subcutaneous reservoir
    - Reservoir is attached to a catheter containing a pump with a one-way valve and is threaded subcutaneously to the peritoneal cavity

Shunt Emergencies

- Most children presenting to the ED have been previously diagnosed and treated with insertion of a VP shunt
- Most common emergencies
  - Shunt malfunction
    - Distal obstruction (thrombosis or displacement)
    - Proximal obstruction (particulate matter—tissue or exudate)
    - Tubing disconnection
    - Migration of distal tip
    - Kinking of the catheter
    - Signs of acute shunt malfunction in infants (increasing ICP)

- Increasing head circumference
- Bulging or tenseness of fontanels
- Separation of suture lines
- Changes in behavior/feeding
- Irritability
- Lethargy
- Vomiting
- Seizures
- Signs of acute shunt malfunction in older children (increasing intracranial pressure [ICP])
  - Change in level of consciousness (LOC)
  - Change in behavior/interaction with environment
  - Vomiting
  - Headache
  - Ataxia
  - Strabismus
  - Seizures
- Specific diagnostic studies
  - "Shunt series"—plain radiographic views of lateral neck, chest, and abdomen to determine position of catheter tip in abdomen, integrity of shunt, and length of catheter remaining
  - CT scan for visualization of ventricular size and signs of increased ICP
  - Pumping of the catheter reservoir is not recommended as a reliable assessment of shunt function
  - Access to the shunt reservoir to measure CSF pressure (recommend consultation with neurosurgeon)
- Disposition
  - Prepare for admission and/or surgery for shunt revision
  - Admission to pediatric ICU for stabilization of increased ICP prior to surgery dependent on severity of condition
- Shunt infection

- May occur at any time—greatest risk, 1–2 mo after insertion
- May include
  - Ascending infection following perforation of bowel by distal catheter tip
  - Meningitis
  - Ventriculitis
- Symptoms
  - Nausea
  - Headache
  - Fever (may be minimal)
  - Malaise, lethargy
  - Altered LOC
- Cultures of CSF may be obtained from shunt reservoir (recommend consultation with neurosurgeon)
- Treatment and disposition
  - Massive doses of antibiotics (IV or intra-ventricular) begun in ED
  - Admission to pediatric ICU or transfer
  - Shunt removal usually required
  - External ventricular drainage until CSF is sterile
  - Referral of family to
    National Hydrocephalus Foundation
    Route 1, River Road
    Box 210A
    Joliet, IL 60436

MENINGITIS

- Acute inflammation of the meninges, membranes that surround brain and spinal column
  - Continued inflammation leads to increased ICP with subdural empyema
  - Continued infection can reach the ventricles
  - CSF is good medium for bacterial growth
  - White blood cells (WBC) are not able to function as defense mechanism against infection in CSF
    - Infection progresses rapidly

- • Changes in permeability of capillaries and blood vessels in dura mater
  - • Increased leakage of albumin and water into subdural space
    - • Further increases in ICP
- • Types of meningitis
  - • Bacterial (Tables 10–2 and 10–3)
    - • Organisms usually spread via droplet transmission, colonize nasopharynx, and spread via bloodstream to meninges
    - • Organisms may be introduced into CNS

Table 10–2. Common Causative Organisms of Bacterial Meningitis

Age of Child	Common Cause	Empiric Antibiotic Treatment*
0–1 mo	Group B streptococcus Escherichia coli Listeria monocytogenes	Cefotaxime and ampicillin $\pm$ gentamicin
1–3 mo	Neisseria meningitidis Haemophilus influenzae type b (Hib) Streptococcus pneumoniae Group B streptococcus E. coli L. monocytogenes	Cefotaxime and ampicillin
3 mo–5 yr	N. meningitidis H. influenzae type b (Hib) S. pneumoniae	Ceftriaxone or cefotaxime
≥6 yr	N. meningitidis S. pneumoniae	Ceftriaxone or cefotaxime

From Davies E, Elliman D, Hart C, et al: Manual of Childhood Infections. Philadelphia, W.B. Saunders, 1996.
*Note: Chloramphenicol and penicillin G also may be used.

Table 10–3. Signs and Symptoms of Bacterial Meningitis

Neonate	Infant-Toddler	Preschooler-Adolescent
Symptoms often vague	Poor feeds	Loss of appetite
Poor feeds	Vomiting	Headache
Weak suck	Fever (may be absent in young infant)	Fever
Weak cry	Ataxia	Myalgias
Poor muscle tone	Lethargy	Vomiting and diarrhea
Irritability	Irritability	Photophobia
Fever or hypothermia	High-pitched cry	Meningeal signs:
Vomiting or diarrhea	Alteration in LOC	+ Kernig's sign (pain with extension of leg and knee)
Irregular breathing patterns	Bulging fontanelle	+ Brudzinski's sign (flexion of head resulting in flexion of hips and knees)
Apnea	Petechia or purpura	+ Nuchal rigidity
Alteration in level of consciousness	*Meningeal signs may be absent in child <2 yr	Confusion
Bulging or tense fontanelle		Alteration in level of consciousness
Opisthotonus		Seizures
Seizures		Purpura
Petechia or purpura		
*Meningeal signs may be absent		

177

by trauma, neurosurgery, or via systemic infection
- Viral
- Vaccination for *Haemophilus influenzae* type b (Hib) is recommended for all children beginning at 2 mo of age
  - Declining incidence of this disease is attributed to the introduction of the Hib vaccine
- Signs and symptoms may vary
  - Limited to fever, stiff neck, and headache
  - Inclusive of previously cited symptoms associated with bacterial meningitis
- Diagnostic studies
  - CBC with differential
  - Serum chemistry profile
    - Including glucose, protein, electrolytes
  - Coagulation profile for suspected disseminated intravascular coagulation (DIC)
  - Blood culture and sensitivity
  - Urinalysis and urine culture and sensitivity
  - Urine osmolarity (will be increased with increased secretion of antidiuretic hormone
  - CT if increased ICP is suspected
  - Lumbar puncture (LP)
    - If delay encountered in performing LP, *do not delay administration of antibiotics*
    - Send CSF obtained after antibiotic therapy has begun for identification of bacterial antigens by latex agglutination or counterimmunophoresis
    - CSF analysis (Table 10–4) includes
      - Cell count and differential
      - Glucose, protein, lactate
      - Bacterial and viral cultures
      - Gram stain

ED treatment
- ABCs
- Initiate respiratory isolation and maintain for 24 hr after antibiotics have been started

Table 10–4. CSF Results in Bacterial vs. Viral Meningitis

	Bacterial	Viral
WBCs	Increased (2000–20,000 μL)	<500 μL
Glucose	Decreased compared with blood glucose	Normal
Protein	Increased	Normal or minimally increased
Gram stain	Bacteria present	No bacteria
Lactate	Increased	Normal

- Maintain patent airway, anticipate intubation if condition warrants
- Administer high concentration oxygen, in method tolerated by child
- Initiate IV access for initial blood draw, administration of fluids, antibiotics, and other medications
  - Anticipate IV fluid bolus of 20 mL/kg of crystalloid solution for hypotension, poor perfusion
    - Repeat bolus as necessary
    - If no response to fluid boluses, anticipate vasopressors and inotropes for septic shock
    - IV fluids given at maintenance rate for stable child
  - Anticipate fluid restriction (60–70% maintenance) only for child with signs of syndrome of inappropriate antidiuretic hormone (SIADH)
    - SIADH
      - Hyponatremia (<130 mmol/L)
      - Urine sodium >60 mmol/L
      - Urine specific gravity >1.020
      - Serum osmolarity <275 mOsm/L
      - Urine osmolarity >300 mOsm/L

- Administer antipyretics for fever—maintain normothermia
- Administer pain relief medication
- Administer dexamethasone IV (0.6 mg/kg/day)
  - For suspected *H. influenzae* meningitis
  - Reduces the incidence of subsequent hearing loss
    - Frequent to continuous monitoring of cardiorespiratory and neurologic status
  - Vital signs with temperature
  - Intake and output with frequent assessments for fluid overload
  - Urinary catheter
  - Consider nasogastric or orogastric tube
  - Modified (pediatric) Glasgow Coma Score (GCS)
  - Pupillary reaction
  - Initiate seizure precautions
- Prepare the child (and family) for diagnostic testing with age-appropriate explanations
- Identify close exposures for possible prophylaxis
  - Positive identification of *Neisseria meningitidis*
  - Rifampin PO may be prescribed for contacts
- Encourage family to participate in care as able
- ED treatment of viral meningitis is mainly symptomatic and comfort measures
  - Usually self-limiting
- Disposition
  - Admission or transfer to pediatric ICU
    - Unstable cardiorespiratory status
    - Elevated ICP
    - Status epilepticus
    - Decreased LOC, coma
  - Admission to pediatric unit for close observation
  - Maintain respiratory isolation

MENINGOCOCCEMIA

- May occur with or without meningitis
- Incubation: 2–10 days
- Presence of *N. meningitidis* in blood
- Signs and symptoms
  - Fever (or hypothermia in neonate, young infant)
  - Headache
  - Irritability
  - Altered LOC
  - Rash—petechia, purpura
- Prognosis poor, as shock and DIC occur quickly

CEREBRAL PALSY (CP)

- Nonprogressive neurologic disorder
- Characterized by impaired movement and posture
- Causes
  - Prenatal
  - Perinatal
  - Postnatal
- Five classifications
  - Athetoid or dyskinetic
    - Uncontrolled, involuntary movements of all extremities
  - Spastic
    - Hypertonicity, increased deep tendon reflexes
    - Stimulus can cause sudden jerking movements
  - Ataxic
    - Disintegration of movements, appears clumsy
  - Rigid or atonic
    - Rigidity in flexor and extensor muscles
    - Associated with multiple deformities because of limited movement
  - Mixed

- • Combination of spasticity
- Disabilities associated with CP
  - Mental retardation
    - May have normal IQ and only appear retarded
  - Learning disabilities, developmental delays
  - Hyperactivity
  - Hearing or visual impairments
  - Gastroesophageal reflux
  - Dysphagia
  - Seizures
  - Joint contractures, dislocations
  - Perceptual deficits
- Children previously diagnosed with CP seen in the ED
  - Trauma caused by spasms, uncontrolled movements, and seizures
    - Head trauma, contusions, lacerations, sprains
    - Assess for possible child maltreatment
      - Higher risk of maltreatment associated with caring for disabled children
  - Seizures
  - Respiratory infection caused by immobility and aspiration pneumonia
  - Surface trauma and skin ulcerations from
    - Splints and braces
    - Poor nutrition
    - Spasticity and immobility

ED treatment
- Based on presenting complaint
- Do not remove braces or body jacket until cervical spine or other fractures have been ruled out
- Maintain safe environment, prevent injury
  - Keep side rails in up position at all times
  - Remove equipment and items that could cause injury from immediate area
  - Seizure precautions as indicated
  - Aspiration precautions as indicated

- • Prevent unnecessary pressure on bony prominences
- • Reposition frequently
- Do not "talk down" to child
- Involve parents in child's care
  - Calming effect on child
  - Facilitate communication—verbal and non-verbal
  - Suggestions and assistance with oral medication administration
- Provide psychosocial and emotional support for parents
  - Stress of caring for chronically ill child is often overwhelming
  - Offer resources:
    United Cerebral Palsy
    1660 L Street, NW Suite 700
    Washington, DC 20036
    800-872-5827
    Fax: 800-776-0414
    e-mail: ucpnatl@ucpa.org

MYELOMENINGOCELE

- Congenital neural tube defect
- Referred to as spina bifida
- Meningocele—an exterior sac with spinal fluid and meninges
- Myelomeningocele—exterior sac with spinal fluid, meninges, nerve roots, and spinal cord
- Degree of muscular weakness or paralysis is dependent on level of defect
- Children presenting to ED with myelomeningocele have already been diagnosed and may have undergone one or more surgical procedures related to the defect
- Children presenting to the ED with myelomeningocele
  - Complaints related to hydrocephalus
    - Hydrocephalus is present in 80% of children with myelomeningocele
    - Refer to previous section on shunt malfunction

- Complaints related to immobility
  - Skin ulcerations
  - Respiratory infections
  - Phlebitis, thrombosis
- Complaints related to diminished or absent sensation in lower extremities
  - Surface trauma, burns, fractures
- Complaints related to neurogenic bladder and bowel
  - Urinary tract infection (UTI), pyleonephritis
  - Constipation, bowel obstruction
- Allergic reactions
  - Particularly to latex
    - Repeated latex exposures during multiple surgeries and invasive procedures
    - 18–60% of children with spina bifida have latex allergy

ED treatment
- Based on presenting complaint
- Do *not* remove braces from child until cervical spine and/or other fractures have been ruled out
- Implement latex precautions, even if previously nonreactive
- Maintain safe environment, prevent injury
  - Side rails in raised position at all times
  - Prevent unnecessary pressure on lower body
    - Reposition frequently
- Prepare for diagnostic procedures and interventions
  - Use age-appropriate explanations
    - Lumbar puncture
    - CT scan and other radiology studies
    - Enemas
    - Urinary catheterization
- Involve parents in child's care
- Provide psychosocial and emotional support to the parents
  - Stress of caring for a chronically ill child is often overwhelming

- Referrals and resources:
Spina Bifida Association of America
800-621-3141
Fax: (202) 944-3295
e-mail: sbaa@sbaa.org
- Discharge instructions
  - Reinforcement of bladder training
    - Diet modifications for bladder control
    - Prevention of UTI
  - Reinforcement of bowel training
    - High-fiber diet, bulking agents
    - Stool softeners
    - Digital stimulation

HEAD TRAUMA

- Trauma is the number-one cause of death in children <18 yr
- Head injury is the leading cause of traumatic death and disability in children
- Head injuries are uncommon in infants <1 yr
  - Evaluate for signs of child maltreatment
- Pediatric considerations in head injury
  - Head is disproportionately larger than body size
  - Neck muscles are weak; ligaments are lax
  - Brain is more fragile
  - Cranium is thinner—less protection to brain
  - Anterior fontanel closes by 18 mo
  - Posterior fontanel closes by 2 mo
  - Brain weight at birth is 60% of adult brain weight
    - By 6 yr, 90% of adult brain weight
  - Decreased autoregulation in children <1 yr because of immaturity of brain
  - Brain has more water, less subarachnoid space than in adult
    - Less CSF to act as a cushion
      - CSF volume in infant = 50 mL; in adult = 150 mL
    - Nerves not completely myelinated at birth—slower conduction of impulses

Traumatic Brain Injury (TBI) Pathophysiology

- TBI types
  - Contusion—localized lesions
  - Hematoma—subdural, epidural, parenchymal
    - Decreased incidence of hematoma in children <5 yr
  - Ischemic injury—associated with high incidence of mortality
  - Axonal injury—local or diffuse
- Severe TBI associated with Glasgow Coma Score of ≤8
- Primary insult of TBI is the injury that occurs at time of impact
  - Secondary insult occurs as the consequence of initial injury
    - Cerebral ischemia→hypoxia→hypercapnia→hypotension→increased ICP
- Brain has a high requirement for oxygen; 20% of total oxygen available to body
- Cerebral blood flow (CBF) is controlled by cerebral perfusion pressure (CPP)
  - CPP = mean arterial pressure (MAP) − ICP
- Cerebral hyperemia—increased CBF with resultant brain swelling
- Cerebral edema—increased water content of brain; may result from ischemia or hypoxia
- Autoregulation—cerebral arteries have ability to change diameter in response to CPP
  - Maintains adequate CBF with changes in blood pressure (BP) and perfusion
  - Ischemia and trauma will impair autoregulation
  - Affected by changes in $Paco_2$ and Pao_2
    - Decreased $Paco_2$ (<25–30 mm Hg) will cause cerebral vasoconstriction, which decreases CBF
    - Decreased Pao_2 (<80 mm Hg) results in increased CBF

- Monroe-Kellie doctrine—to maintain cerebral pressure and cerebral volume in a normal range; a change in one or more cranial contents will result in a change in another cranial content
  - Cranial contents: blood, brain tissue, CSF
  - Compensation for an abnormal change occurs by
    - Decreased CSF production
    - Increased CSF absorption
    - Reduction in cerebral mass by fluid displacement
  - Compensation is time limited (can occur for only so long)
    - Any other increase in volume or pressure will result in a sudden increase in ICP
    - The increase in ICP will result in
      - Decreased perfusion, which causes a shift in brain tissue, resulting in herniation
      - Death usually results from pressure on the brain stem
- Coup-contrecoup injuries (Fig. 10–1)
  - Acceleration-deceleration injury
  - Shearing forces result in bruising, tearing, bleeding

Assessment

- General assessment
  - Assessment of ABCs; maintain cervical spine immobilization (see also Section III, Chapter 15 Trauma)
  - Complete history
    - MIVT assessment tool
      - **M**echanism and pattern of injury
      - **I**njuries suspected
      - **V**ital signs
        - Important to ascertain if even a single hypotensive episode has occurred since time of injury
          - Associated with a poorer outcome

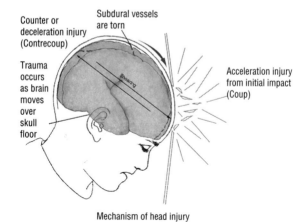

Mechanism of head injury

Figure 10–1. Mechanism of head injury. (From Ashwill J, Droske S: Nursing Care of Children: Principles and Practice. Philadelphia, W.B. Saunders, 1997, p. 1260.)

- **T**reatment initiated and patient responses (prehospital)
- CIAMPEDS (see Section I, Reference 27, CIAMPEDS Triage History)
- Assess for possible cervical spine injury or SCIWORA (see "Spinal Trauma")
- Ongoing continued assessments
  - Vital signs
  - LOC
    - AVPU assessment tool
      - **A**lert
      - **V**erbal—responds to verbal stimuli
      - **P**ain—responds to painful stimuli
      - **U**nresponsive
    - Pediatric or modified GCS (see Section I, Reference 13, Pediatric Modification of Glasgow Coma Scale by Age of Patient)
      - Record and report GCS as follows
        - Eye = __
        - Verbal = __
        - Motor = __
        - Total GCS = __

- Oxygenation—pulse oximetry, capnography
- Pupillary size and reaction
- Intake and output
- Signs and symptoms are related to mechanism of injury (MOI) and subsequent increase in ICP

Selected Head Trauma Emergencies

Surface trauma

- Lacerations
- Abrasions
- Bleeding
- Subgaleal hematoma

Skull fractures

- Linear
  - Most common
  - No involvement of dura
  - Temporal bone is the weakest bone
    - Risk of epidural bleeding if fracture is over middle meningeal artery
    - Frequently associated with vomiting
- Depressed
  - Skull fragment intrudes into cranial vault
  - Pressure placed on brain
  - Often palpable
- Basilar
  - Fracture at the base of skull
    - Frontal, ethmoid, sphenoid, temporal, or occipital bones
  - Signs and symptoms
    - Changes in LOC or behavior
      - Irritability, agitation
    - CSF leakage from ear or nose
      - Halo or ring sign
        - Check for presence of CSF in bloody drainage by placing one drop on filter paper (or white cloth); formation of one

or more clear rings indicates presence of CSF
  • May also check for presence of glucose in clear drainage
    • Presence of glucose indicates presence of CSF
• Periorbital ecchymosis—"raccoon's eyes" (seen 12–24 hr after injury)
• Ecchymosis of mastoid area—"Battle's sign"
  • Blood collects in mastoid air cells
  • Usually seen 12–24 hr after injury
• Hemotympanum blood behind the tympanic membrane

Concussion

• Characterized by temporary loss of consciousness, except in very young children, in whom
  • Loss of consciousness not common
  • Sleepiness and vomiting more frequent
  • Postinjury seizures are common

Contusion

• Bruise on the brain with microscopic hemorrhage
• Often associated with coup-contrecoup MOI (see Fig. 10–1) or blunt injury
• Signs and symptoms vary with location and size of lesions
  • Alteration in LOC
  • Nausea, vomiting
  • Visual defects
  • Weakness
  • Speech defects
• Severe contusions may result in intracerebral hemorrhage
• Prepare for CT scan
• Prepare for surgery if substantial hemorrhage and neurologic deficits

Hematoma

• Epidural—bleeding between the skull and the dura mater

- More common in older children
- May be associated with skull fracture and injury to middle meningeal artery
- Signs and symptoms
  - 20–25% of children will have a transient loss of consciousness followed by alertness, then a repeated loss of consciousness
  - Decreased LOC
  - Headache
  - Contralateral hemiparesis
  - Fixed and dilated pupil on same side as injury
- CT scan—biconvex area of density
- Interventions include continuous monitoring and repeated assessments (see section on general assessment)
  - Prepare for surgery
- Subdural—bleeding into space between dura and arachnoid membrane
  - Bridging vessels between cerebral cortex and dura are torn
  - More frequent than epidural hematoma
  - Commonly associated with shaken impact syndrome, falls, motor vehicle crashes
  - Signs and symptoms
    - Altered LOC
    - Loss of consciousness since injury
    - Infants: bulging fontanel
    - Lethargy, irritability, coma
    - Increased deep tendon reflexes (DTRs)
    - Positive Babinski sign
  - CT scan
    - Increased density over entire cerebral cortex
    - Edema at site of injury
    - Midline shift seen with significant brain injury
  - Disposition—will require admission or transfer to a pediatric ICU
    - Older child—surgical intervention often necessary

- Infant—subdural taps (most often performed in the ICU) to remove fluid and thus decrease ICP
- Parenchymal—brain lacerations
  - May produce significant blood loss
  - Signs and symptoms dependent on area of injury and associated injuries

Ischemic injury

- Infarction of brain
- Associated with poor outcome
- Identified in 90% of fatal head injuries
- Injured brain susceptible to hypoxic-ischemic insults
  - Moderate levels of hypoxia, usually well tolerated in noninjured brain, may induce permanent damage in the injured brain
  - Even one documented hypotensive episode has been correlated with a poorer outcome

Axonal injury

- Stretching or transection of axons by shearing forces
- Usual cause is rotational acceleration-deceleration injury
- Local or diffuse
- Diffuse axonal injury (DAI)
  - Sustained coma after injury
  - Seizures common
  - No mass lesion on CT or MRI
  - Mild—loss of consciousness: 6–24 hr
    - Improvement after 24 hr
  - Moderate—coma: >24 hr
    - Posturing indicative of brain stem dysfunction
  - Severe—coma for days or weeks
    - Autonomic dysfunction: hyperthermia, hypertension, diaphoresis
    - Poor prognosis

General Interventions for the Child With a Head Injury

- Stabilize ABCs
  - Airway—secure airway in children with a total GCS of ≤8
    - Rapid-sequence intubation for a child with a head injury
      - Preoxygenation with 100%
      - Fentanyl 1–2 μg/kg IV
      - Diazepam or midazolam 0.1–0.3 mg/kg IV
      - Vecuronium 0.2–0.3 mg/kg IV
      - Cricoid pressure
    - In the presence of impending herniation—immediate intubation
      - Thiopental 5–7 mg/kg IV
      - Lidocaine 1 mg/kg IV
      - Vecuronium 0.2–0.3 mg/kg IV
  - Maintain cervical spine immobilization, discontinue only after
    - Full cervical spine series has been cleared
    - Child has no evidence of neurologic deficits
  - Breathing—maintain PaO_2 at ≥90 mm Hg
  - Obtain IV access for fluid and medication administration
    - Fluid resuscitation for decreased BP
      - A single hypotensive episode is associated with a poorer outcome
      - CPP = ICP − MAP
        - A decrease in volume will decrease CPP
    - Maintenance fluids to produce a urine output of 1–2 ml/kg/hr and serum sodium of 135–145 mEq/L
- Ongoing continuous monitoring and assessment
  - ABCs
  - Vital signs
  - Neurologic status
    - Pupillary size and reaction

- • GCS
- • Intake and output
- • Pulse oximetry, capnography, cardiac rhythm, noninvasive BP or intraarterial BP
- • Elevate head of bed 30° when cervical spine immobilization has been discontinued
  - • Facilitate jugular venous drainage and possibly CSF drainage without a negative effect on CPP
- • Maintain normothermia
  - • Every 1°C rise in temperature is accompanied by a 13% rise in metabolism
- • Observe closely for Cushing's response (Cushing's triad)
  - • A late sign in a young child
  - • Indicates an increasing ICP
    - • Normal ICP = 0–10 mm Hg
  - • Elevated BP is a compensatory attempt to perfuse the brain
  - • Decreased heart rate
  - • Decreased respiratory rate or apnea
- • Initiate measure to monitor, control, and decrease ICP
  - • Intracranial hypertension = ICP >20 mm Hg for >5 min
  - • Elevated ICP >3–4 hr associated with a poorer outcome
  - • Consider *early* transfer to a pediatric ICU
  - • Monitoring ICP
    - • Recommended with TBI and GCS ≤ 8 and no spontaneous eye opening
    - • Variety of ICP monitoring devices available
      - • Subarachnoid bolt most common in ED setting
      - • Intraventricular catheter is the device of choice
        - • Placed in ICU or surgery
        - • Able to monitor ICP and remove excess fluid from ventricles
  - • Interventions to decrease ICP
    - • Position with head of bed at 30°

- Ventilation
  - Prophylactic hyperventilation ($Paco_2$ = 22–30 mm Hg) is of *no* benefit and may be associated with a poorer outcome
  - Normocarbia and hypercarbia are *not* recommended
  - *Mild* hyperventilation is recommended ($Paco_2$ = 30–35 mm Hg)
  - Hyperventilation is used only at impending herniation
- Mannitol
  - Decreases blood viscosity, resulting in decreased cerebral blood volume
    - No change in CBF
    - Transient decrease in ICP
    - Autoregulation must be intact
  - Osmotic process results in dehydrating effect
    - Blood-brain barrier must be intact
  - Dose: 0.25 or 0.50 g/kg/dose over 10–15 min
    - Administered every 6 hr as needed
    - May repeat dose as necessary for intracranial hypertension
    - Contraindicated if serum osmolality >330 mmol/L
- Barbiturates
  - Decreases ICP by decreasing cerebral metabolism
    - Produces a decrease in CBF and a decrease in cerebral blood volume
  - Also demonstrate neuroprotectant effects
  - Used in refractory intracranial hypertension
    - ICU setting with monitoring of EEG to assess response to treatment
  - *Must* avoid hypotension
  - Loading dose
    - Pentobarbital or thiopental: ~30 mg/kg over 3 hr
    - Intermittent doses of 3–5 mg/kg

- Temperature
  - Maintain normothermia
    - Induced hypothermia is a last resort
- BP
  - When autoregulation no longer functions, CBF is directly related to CPP
    - Decrease in BP will result in a decrease in CBF
  - When autoregulation remains intact
    - Decrease in BP results in a decrease in CPP
    - Reflex cerebral vasodilation will increase the cerebral blood volume and increase the ICP

Disposition—Varies With the Severity of the Injury

- Observation at home by caregivers
  - GCS of 14 or greater, minor trauma, normal CT scan
  - Discharge instructions include when to call physician or return to the ED
    - Seizure activity
    - Confusion, change in personality
    - Severe headache
    - Difficulty awakening
    - Vomiting more than three times
    - Blurred vision, slurred speech
    - Unequal pupils
    - Difficulty walking or crawling
    - Weakness of extremities
  - Discuss light diet and limitation of activities at home
- Hospitalization
  - Prolonged loss of consciousness
  - Coma, altered LOC, seizures
  - Focal neurologic deficits
  - Persistent vomiting
  - Severe headache
  - Alcohol or drug intoxication

- Suspected child maltreatment
- Transfer/admission to a pediatric ICU
  - Severe TBI
  - Requires ICP monitoring or ventilator support

SPINAL TRAUMA

- Rare in children
- Fracture of vertebral bodies
- Subluxation of vertebrae
  - Malalignment of contiguous vertebrae
    - Compression of spinal cord
      - Spinal cord may be crushed, over-stretched, or severed
- Most often associated with multisystem trauma
  - Falls, jumps
  - Motor vehicle crashes
  - Sports activities
    - Diving, surfing, swimming
  - Child maltreatment
  - Penetrating trauma
    - Gunshot wounds
  - Hanging
- Pediatric considerations
  - Head is disproportionately larger
    - Head, rather than neck, is often the site of injury
    - Be suspicious of cervical spine injury with associated head injury
    - Neck ligaments are lax, highly elastic
      - Allows for more movement with less bony injury
  - Bony spine is similar to adult spine by 8–10 yr
    - Child <8 yr has greater risk for higher cervical spine injury (C3–C4)
  - Spinal cord injury without radiographic abnormality (SCIWORA)
    - Syndrome characterized by no visual deformity or bony injury on x-ray or CT scan
    - Myelogram may be needed for diagnosis

- Child presents with either complete or incomplete spinal cord syndromes
- May have delayed onset of symptoms

Signs and Symptoms
- Pain with palpation over spinal column
- Poikilothermia—assumes temperature of surroundings
- Weakness or paralysis in extremities
- Paresthesias
- Loss of sphincter tone

History
- MIVT (see "Head Trauma")
- CIAMPEDS (see Section I, Reference 27, CIAMPEDS Triage History)
- Child's description of neck pain at any time after injury
- Changes in sensation or movement since injury
- If a fall, was it greater than three times the child's height?
- Loss of bladder or bowel control in the toilet-trained child

Diagnostic Studies
- Cross-table lateral cervical spine x-ray
  - Must visualize all seven cervical vertebrae and the C7–T1 junction
- Cervical spine series (cross-table, anteroposterior, odontoid views)
  - Swimmer's view may be necessary to view cervical vertebrae
  - Open-mouth series may be necessary to view odontoid body, C1, and C2
- CT scan
- MRI
  - Used in conjunction with CT scan, may be useful in SCIWORA
- Myelogram—especially useful in SCIWORA

ED Treatment
- ABCs
- Maintain cervical spine immobilization
  - <10 yr—use a spine board with a recessed area for the child's occiput
  - Manual stabilization initially, followed by definitive stabilization
    - Use rolled towels, other padding, rigid cervical collars in appropriate size
    - Tape head to board
    - Place straps across body at chest, abdomen, and knees
- Administration of steroids—methylprednisolone
  - Decrease edema
  - Anti-inflammatory
  - Protect cell membrane by scavenging oxygen free radicals
  - Dose
    - Initial IV bolus within 8 hr of injury
      - 30 mg/kg over 15 min
    - 45 min later, begin infusion of 5.4 mg/kg/hr for 23 hr
- Insert indwelling urinary catheter
- Insert oral or nasal gastric tube
- Maintain normothermia
  - Initiate heat measures
    - Blankets, overhead lights, warmed IV fluids
- Continued assessment
  - Vital signs
  - Heart rate and rhythm
  - Oxygen saturation
  - Pediatric GCS
    - Record and report according to E, V, M (see Head Trauma)
  - AVPU (LOC)—(see Head Trauma)

Complete spinal cord injury

- Spinal shock
  - Loss of motor and sensory function below level of injury

- Injuries usually above T6
- Signs and symptoms
  - Flaccid paralysis
  - Loss of sphincter tone
  - Bradycardia
    - Bounding peripheral pulses
  - Hypotension
  - Cool, dry skin
- Must quickly assess for other causes of shock (e.g., intra-abdominal hemorrhage)

Incomplete spinal cord injury

- Central cord syndrome—loss of function in upper extremities only
- Anterior cord syndrome—hyperesthesia, hypoalgesia, incomplete or complete paralysis
- Posterior cord syndrome
- Brown-Séquard syndrome
  - Most common with penetrating trauma
  - Ipsilateral motor and proprioception loss
  - Contralateral pain and temperature deficit
  - May be seen with or without fracture

Autonomic dysreflexia

- Complication of injuries above level of T6
- Various stimuli may trigger autonomic dysreflexia
  - Full bladder or rectum
  - Decubitus ulcer
  - Stimuli causes the sympathetic nervous system to overreact
- Signs and symptoms
  - Severe headache
  - Sweating
  - Nasal stuffiness
  - Tachycardia or bradycardia
  - Flushing above injury/coolness below injury
  - Anxiety

ED treatment
- Assess for possible stimulus and remove it
  - For example, removal of occluded urinary catheter and insertion of new patent catheter
- Administer ganglionic blockers
  - Hydralazine (Apresoline), diazoxide (Hyperstat), nifedipine (Procardia), atropine

Disposition

- All children with spinal cord injury are transferred or admitted to a pediatric and/or neurologic ICU or spinal cord injury ICU

Prevention

- Encourage use of helmets, seat belts, and other safety devices
- Review with parents
  - Correct (safest) placement of children in a vehicle
  - Proper installation of an infant or child car seat in a vehicle
- Discuss risky sports and behaviors with children at appropriate developmental level
  - Use of alcohol or other substances
  - Snowboarding
  - Diving

Selected Bibliography

Ashwill JW, Droske SC: Nursing Care of Children: Principles and Practice. Philadelphia, W.B. Saunders, 1997.

Barkin R, Rosen P: Emergency Pediatrics: A Guide to Ambulatory Care, 4th ed. St. Louis, Mosby–Year Book, 1994.

Haley K, Baker P (eds): Instructor Manual: Emergency Nursing Pediatric Course. Chicago, Emergency Nurses Association, 1993.

Klinkhammer B, Andreoni C: Quick Reference for Emergency Nursing. Philadelphia, W.B. Saunders, 1998.

Newberry L (ed): Sheehy's Emergency Nursing: Principles and Practice, 4th ed. St. Louis, Mosby–Year Book, 1998.

Singh N: Manual of Pediatric Critical Care. Philadelphia, W.B. Saunders, 1977.

Soud TE, Rogers JS: Manual of Pediatric Emergency Nursing. St. Louis, Mosby–Year Book, 1998.

Chapter 11
Orthopedic

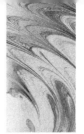

SEPTIC ARTHRITIS

- An infection of the joint space
- Usually caused by bacterial pathogens
  - Hematogenous spread from distal site of infection
    - Otitis media
    - Upper respiratory infection
    - Puncture wound contamination
    - Cellulitis
    - Osteomyelitis
- Usually seen in infants and children up to age 2 yr, and during adolescence
  - <1 yr of age, capillaries perforate growth plate
    - Infection can spread across the epiphysis
  - >5 yr of age, infection, trauma, or both are prime causes
- Can result in necrosis of the epiphysis and growth plate, destruction of joint capsule and ligaments

Signs and Symptoms

- Fever and/or chills
- Erythema of the joint
- Inability to tolerate active or passive range of motion (ROM) of joint
- Palpable joint effusion
  - Harder to detect in hip joint
- Symptoms generally have an acute onset but can be slower
- Infants may have symptoms noted during routine diaper change
- Toddlers and children may limp

Emergency Department (ED) Treatment

- Complete blood count (CBC), erythrocyte sedimentation rate (ESR), blood culture(s)
- Arthrocentesis (test of choice for rapid diagnosis)
- Potassium hydroxide preparation for fungi in neonates or immunosuppressed patients
- X-rays to rule out osteomyelitis
- Vaginal, rectal, pharyngeal cultures to rule out *Neisseria gonorrhoeae* infection
- IV access
  - IV antibiotic therapy
- Hospital admission

OSTEOMYELITIS

- Infection of the bones
- Usually caused by bacterial pathogens
  - Hematogenous spread from distal site of infection
    - Puncture wounds through tennis shoes
    - Open fractures
    - Contiguous infectious processes (less common in children)
    - Trauma
- Involves rapidly growing bones
- Arteries supply nutrients to growth plates
  - Arterial flow obstructed by bacterial microemboli
  - Results in avascular necrosis and metaphyseal abscess
- Occurs at any age but is common in ages 3–12 yr
  - Boys twice as frequently affected as girls

Signs and Symptoms

- Fever
- Focal bone pain

- • Tenderness
- • Erythema
- Acute onset
- Pseudoparalysis (unwillingness to move limb or bear weight)
- Vertebral site has insidious onset
  - • Backache
  - • Vague symptoms
- Hip/pelvic sites may result in a limp
  - • Abdominal pain
  - • Hip pain
  - • Groin pain

ED Treatment

- CBC, ESR, blood culture(s)
- Tuberculosis skin test (in chronic cases)
- X-rays of affected area and chest
  - • Chest film to rule out *Mycobacterium tuberculosis*
  - • In affected areas, look for
    - • Periosteal elevation
    - • Calcification
    - • Bone destruction
- Wound culture or bone aspiration
- IV access
  - • IV antibiotic therapy
- Extremity immobilization
- Pain control
- Possible surgery to drain area or remove necrotic bone
- Counsel parents/caregiver
  - • Need for high-calorie diet
  - • Fracture risks

TRANSIENT SYNOVITIS

- Inflammation and hypertrophy of synovial membrane of the hip joint
  - • Small synovial effusion is not uncommon
- Etiology is unclear

- Possible links
  - Recent infection
  - Viral illness
  - Trauma
- Children ages 3–8 yr most affected

Signs and Symptoms

- Acute groin pain
- Nontraumatic knee or thigh pain
- A limp in ambulatory children
- Hip may be flexed, abducted, and externally rotated if a significant effusion is present
- Usually afebrile or low-grade fever

ED Treatment

- CBC, ESR
- X-rays
  - Anteroposterior (AP) and lateral frog-leg views of pelvis
- Ultrasound of hip
  - May show a hip joint effusion
- Bone scan
  - Differentiates a septic process
    - Must be identified promptly
- Pain control
  - Nonsteroidal anti-inflammatory drugs (NSAIDs)
- Bedrest with no weight bearing until pain-free
  - Symptoms may exacerbate with too early a return to activity

LEGG-CALVÉ-PERTHES DISEASE (LCPD)

- Avascular necrosis of the capital femoral epiphysis (CFE)
- Caused by an interruption in the CFE blood supply
  - Precipitating factors
    - Trauma

- Stress fracture
- Age of clinical onset is 2–12 yr
  - Boys primarily affected
  - Rare in African-Americans and Asians
- See classification of LCPD (Table 11–1)

Signs and Symptoms

- A painless intermittent limp after activity
  - May progress to constant limp
- Hip, groin, knee pain (mild)
- Slow onset of symptoms
- Muscle spasm

ED Treatment

- Hip x-rays to determine
  - Disease progression
  - Sphericity of the femoral head
  - Rule out CFE collapse
- Bone scan or magnetic resonance imaging
  - Helps determine degree of avascularity
- Maintenance of the femoral head within the acetabulum

Table 11–1. Classification of LCPD	
Stages	**Extent of Involvement**
I	Ischemia causes a reduction in the ossific nucleus of the femoral head
II	The femoral head reduces in size and increases in density; necrosis results causing the bone to weaken and die
III	The femoral head collapses and results in superolateral displacement of the femoral head; the avascular bone is reabsorbed
IV	Final healing occurs as new bone is formed through reconstitution and remodeling

- Traction
- Braces
- Surgery
- Bedrest
- ROM exercises

SLIPPED CFE

- Displacement of the proximal femoral epiphysis
  - Causes displacement of femoral head relative to the femoral neck
- Most common adolescent hip disorder
  - Most prevalent in boys, but does occur in girls
    - Obese with delayed skeletal maturation
      - Obesity results in a weakened, obliquely oriented growth plate
    - Tall and thin following a recent growth spurt
- Acute slippage from trauma, chronic disease, or shearing stress from body weight
  - Higher incidence in African-American population
- Can occur in association with endocrine disorders
  - Hypothyroidism
  - Pituitary disorders
  - Recombinant growth hormone therapy
- Both hips affected ~33% of the time
  - Unusual for simultaneous bilateral occurrence

Signs and Symptoms

- Acute
  - Severe hip pain
    - Pain may radiate to groin, thigh, knee
  - External rotation with shortening
- Chronic
  - Slower onset of dull hip pain
    - Dull pain radiates to groin, thigh, knee

- Occasional limp
- Pain increased with activity
- Slight to severe decreased ROM
- Leg may be shortened
- See classification of slipped CFE (Table 11–2)

ED Treatment

- AP and frog-leg x-rays of pelvis
  - Assesses hips for posterior displacement of femoral head
- No weight bearing
- Traction
- Surgery (scheduled) to prevent slippage
  - Internal fixation

Table 11–2. Classification of Slipped Capital Femoral Epiphysis (CFE)

Clinical Group	Description
Preslip	Widened physis, but slippage has not occurred; mild pain; normal physical findings
Acute	Pain, limp for <3 wk; acute and sudden slippage with or without trauma; child cannot bear weight; CFE is *unstable*
Acute-on-chronic	An acute slippage of the CFE on an existing chronic slip; several months of previous symptoms: pain, limp, out-toed gait; trauma is most likely factor contributing to acute slip; CFE is *unstable*
Chronic	Most common type; several months of nonsevere symptoms: pain, limp, out-toed gait; symptoms worsen as the slip progresses; child is able to walk and bear weight; the CFE is *stable*

- Bone grafting
- Osteotomies of femoral neck or subtrochan-teric areas to realign the proximal femur
- Hip spica cast application
  - Cast care instructions to parent/caregiver
- Analgesics

OSGOOD-SCHLATTER DISEASE

- Fibrocartilage microfracture of the tibial tuber-cle at the patellar ligament insertion site
- Occurs during late childhood to early adoles-cence
  - Most common in ages 8–16 yr
  - More common in boys
- Exacerbated by running and jumping activities
- Self-limiting
  - Does not cause permanent damage to the knee joint
    - The patellar ligament and tibial tubercle are extraarticular

Signs and Symptoms

- Anterior aspect knee pain
  - Worsens with activity or direct pressure (kneeling)
- Swelling of the tibial tubercle
- Exquisite pain at the tibial tubercle
- Possible weight-bearing difficulty

ED Treatment

- X-ray to rule out other lesions
  - Diagnosis of Osgood-Schlatter disease may be confirmed by the detection of a prominent, irregular tibial tubercle
  - Bone fragments may also be noted on the radiograph
- Knee immobilization in severe cases
- Pain control with NSAIDs
- Restrict activity for 2–3 wk

FRACTURES

- A break in the continuity of a bone
- Occurs when excessive force or trauma is greater than the strength of the bone
- Described by anatomic location
  - Distal
  - Middle
  - Proximal
  - Intraarticular
  - Head
  - Shaft
  - Base
- Open fracture
  - Break in the bone as well as the integrity of the skin
- Closed fracture
  - The integrity of the skin is intact
- Direction of the fracture line
  - Spiral
    - Fracture twists around the shaft of the bone
    - Results from a twisting force
  - Transverse
    - Fracture is 90° to axis of the bone
    - Results from angulation force or direct trauma
  - Oblique
    - Fracture is 45° to axis of the bone
    - Results from twisting force
  - Comminuted
    - More than one fracture line and more than two fragments (includes segmental and butterfly fractures)
    - Results from severe direct trauma
  - Greenstick
    - Incomplete fracture, seen most commonly in children under 10 yr of age
    - Results from compression force
  - Impacted
    - One bony fragment is driven into another
    - Fracture line may not be clearly visible

- Results from severe trauma
- Epiphyseal
  - Fracture occurs between the bone shaft and the epiphyseal plate
  - Serious injury, as it can alter or inhibit growth
  - See Salter-Harris classification (Table 11–3)

Signs and Symptoms

- Pain with palpation
- Pain with movement
- Crepitus
- May or may not exhibit obvious deformity
- Decreased or limited ROM
- Tingling or burning sensation
  - Suggests neurovascular compromise

Table 11–3. Salter-Harris Classification of Epiphyseal Fractures

Type	Description
I	Epiphysis is completely separated from the metaphysis without fracture
II	Transverse fracture extends through the separated epiphyseal plate, resulting in a triangular fracture
III	The fracture is intraarticular and extends through part of the epiphyseal plate into the joint
IV	The fracture is intraarticular and extends through the epiphyseal plate and through the metaphysis
V	Epiphyseal plate is crushed; can appear to be a type I injury on x-ray; can result in cell death of the growth plate; rare injury

ED Treatment

- Must assess mechanism of injury
  - Suspect child maltreatment if the injury is inconsistent with the stated mechanism of injury
  - Children are generally not good historians
    - May point to painful areas above or below the injury
- Airway, breathing, and circulation (ABCs)
  - 40–60% of children with pelvic fractures also have associated head trauma
  - Blood loss can be significant with pelvic and femur fractures
- Immobilization with frequent assessment of distal neurovascular status
  - Assessment of the five Ps
    - Pain
    - Pulses
    - Paresthesia
    - Paralysis
    - Pallor
- Elevation of the fractured area after immobilization with ice bag (cold pack) application
- X-rays of the affected area to include the joint above and joint below site of injury
- IV access
  - Fluid resuscitation prn
  - Pain management
- Nothing by mouth
- Anticipate possible Bier block (see also Section VII, Procedure 14, Application of Splints) for closed reduction of forearm fracture
- Anticipate possible traction splint application for lower extremity fractures
- Hospitalization
  - Possible surgical intervention

COMPARTMENT SYNDROME

- An increase in pressure on, or volume within, a fascial compartment of an extremity

- Compartments that can be affected
  - Shoulders
  - Upper arms
  - Hands
  - Pelvis
  - Hips
  - Thighs
  - Feet
  - Lower leg and forearm most commonly affected in adolescents and adults
- Compartments most commonly affected in children
  - Interosseous compartments of the hands and feet
  - Volar and dorsal compartments of the forearm
  - Thigh

Contributing Factors

- Bleeding
  - History of hemophilia
- Edema
- Constrictive bandages
- Casts

Signs and Symptoms

- Throbbing pain
- Pain increases with passive muscle stretching
- Elevated compartment pressures (Table 11–4)
- If not treated promptly, results in
  - Complete death of structures within the compartment
  - Volkmann's ischemic contracture

ED Treatment

- ABCs
- Initial and frequent assessment of pulses distal to the injury

Table 11–4. Compartment Pressures

Pressure	Description
>30 mm Hg	Capillary pressure is not sufficient to maintain blood flow to the muscles; results in necrosis; significant muscle damage with sustained pressure for 6–8 hr; compartment is taut and feels hard to the touch; skin blisters may develop
40–60 mm Hg	Muscle and nerve ischemia within the compartment; a pressure of >40 mm Hg warrants surgical decompression; arterial flow is preserved
>60 mm Hg	Arterial flow is occluded; duration of the elevated pressure prior to surgical intervention will determine functional outcome; amputation is a consequence of sustained elevated compartment pressure

- Remove the external compressive force
- Elevate the limb no higher than the level of the patient's heart
- Administer analgesics
- Emergent fasciotomy recommended when compartment pressures are >40 mm Hg

NURSEMAID'S ELBOW

- Subluxation of the annular ligament of the elbow
- Caused by sudden jerk on the extended elbow
  - Child falls when being held by the hand
  - Child is forcefully lifted by the hand
- Very common injury seen in the ED

Signs and Symptoms

- Decreased movement of the arm is a classic symptom
- Hand is usually positioned palm-down
- Pain in the elbow or arm

ED Treatment

- Assess neurovascular status
- Treatment entails reduction of the radial head
  - Pressure is applied over the radial head
  - Hand is moved to a palm-up position
  - "Click" is usually felt as the subluxation is reduced
- X-rays are generally not indicated unless fracture is suspected
- Instruct parent/caregiver on the mechanism of injury
  - Once a subluxation has occurred, there is a higher chance of child having subsequent subluxation

SPRAINS AND STRAINS

Sprain

- Ligament is stretched until it tears
- Occurs when a joint exceeds its normal limits
- A more traumatic injury than a strain

Strain

- Involves muscles or tendons
- Occurs at the point where the muscle attaches to the tendon
- Caused by overstretching

Degree of Injury

- First = minor tear
- Second = partial tear
- Third = complete tear of the ligament

Signs and Symptoms

- Pain at site of injury
- May have deformity and swelling in an extremity injury
- Limited ROM
- May or may not be able to bear weight

ED Treatment

- Assessment of the five Ps (see Fractures)
- X-rays of the affected site
- Pain control
- Immobilization of extremity injury with elastic bandage, rigid padded splint (plaster, fiberglass), or other commercial product (air splint)
- Crutches, as indicated, with gait training
- Discharge instructions to parent/caregiver to include RICE mnemonic
  - **R** = *R*est
  - **I** = *I*ce, application of cold
  - **C** = *C*ompression bandage
  - **E** = *E*levation of joint

DUCHENNE TYPE MUSCULAR DYSTROPHY (MD)

- Sex-linked recessive trait
- Boys predominantly affected
- Mothers are generally asymptomatic carriers
- Incidence is 20–30 cases/100,000 live male births

Signs and Symptoms

- May exhibit
  - Walking delays
  - Stair-climbing delays
  - Frequent falls
  - Inability to run properly
- Calf hypertrophy
- Proximal leg weakness

- Gower sign
  - Child rises from a sitting position by climbing up on legs and body
- Waddling gait
- Pain
- Anxiety
- Complications of Duchenne type MD
  - Pulmonary hypoventilation
    - Pneumonia most frequent consequence
  - Congestive heart failure (CHF)

ED Treatment

- ABCs
- Supportive treatment for patient and parent/caregiver
  - Currently, there is no cure for MD
  - Treat symptoms associated with MD
- Muscle biopsy (generally not done in the ED)
- Serum creatine kinase
  - Elevated early in disease
- Pain control

JUVENILE RHEUMATOID ARTHRITIS

- An autoimmune inflammatory disease
- Etiology unknown
- Classified based on clinical manifestations
  - Pauciarticular disease
    - Involves four or fewer joints
  - Polyarticlar disease
    - Involves five or more joints
  - Systemic-onset disease (least common)
    - Spiking high fevers
    - Erythematous macular rash that comes and goes with fever spikes
    - Joint involvement at onset of symptoms or later
- Incidence is 1.4:10,000
- Onset is between ages 1 and 3 and in early adolescence

Signs and Symptoms

- Chronic arthritis lasting >6 wk
  - Pain
  - Swollen joints
  - Limited ROM
  - Stiffness
- Systemic signs
  - Weakness
  - Fatigue
  - Weight loss
  - Fevers
  - Rash
  - Growth retardation

Complications

- Acute joint inflammation
- Infections
- Cardiac symptoms
  - Chest pain
  - Pericarditis
  - CHF
  - Pericardial effusion
- Pulmonary symptoms
  - Pneumonia
  - Pleural effusion
    - Chest pain
    - Cough
- Ophthalmic symptoms
  - Chronic uveitis
    - Inflammation of the eye (red eye)
    - Poor vision
    - Risk of blindness

ED Treatment

- ABCs
- CBC, ESR, rheumatoid factor, antinuclear antibody (ANA)
- X-rays of affected joints as indicated
- Slit lamp examination

- Pain control
  - NSAIDs, antirheumatic drugs, corticosteroids
- Parent/caregiver support
- Referrals
  - Nutritionist
  - Physical therapy
  - Occupational therapy
  - Arthritis Foundation 800-283-7800

Selected Bibliography

Ashwill J, Droske S: Nursing Care of Children: Principles and Practice. Philadelphia, W.B. Saunders, 1997.

Green N, Swiontkowski M: Skeletal Trauma in Children. Philadelphia, W.B. Saunders, 1998.

Kidd P, Sturt P: Mosby's Emergency Nursing Reference. St. Louis, CV Mosby, 1996.

Soud T, Rogers J: Manual of Pediatric Emergency Nursing. St. Louis, Mosby–Year Book, 1998.

Tipsord-Klinkhammer B, Andreoni C: Quick Reference for Emergency Nursing. Philadelphia, W.B. Saunders, 1998.

Chapter 12
Respiratory

APNEA

- Absence of breathing for >20 sec
- Apnea of infancy (AOI)
  - Apnea in infants of >37 wk gestation
  - Clinical presentation: an apparent life-threatening event (ALTE)
    - Previously referred to as a "near-miss sudden infant death syndrome" (SIDS)
    - Emergency department (ED) presentation of infant: completely normal to cardiopulmonary arrest
    - Caregiver's description includes
      - Apnea
      - Color change
      - Marked change in muscle tone
      - Choking or gagging
  - May be a symptom of other disorders
    - Sepsis
    - Seizures
    - Upper airway abnormalities
    - Gastroesophageal refux disease
    - Hypoglycemia
    - Impaired regulation of feeding or sleep
    - Poisoning
    - Metabolic problem
  - Often no cause is identified; diagnosis remains AOI
  - Peak incidence at 8–14 wk of life
  - Increased risk for SIDS
    - <7% of children with SIDs have history of ALTE
- Diagnostic studies
  - Complete blood count (CBC) with differential and platelet count

- Arterial blood gases (ABGs)
- Serum chemistries
- Chest x-ray (CXR)
- Electrocardiogram
- ED treatment
  - Assist with Basic Life Support (BLS) and Pediatric Advanced Life Support (PALS) resuscitation
  - Provide a neutral thermal environment
  - Continuous cardiorespiratory monitoring
- Disposition
  - Infants with an ALTE are admitted for observation and further evaluation
  - Parents are instructed in infant CPR and apnea monitoring prior to discharge home from the hospital

SUDDEN INFANT DEATH SYNDROME (SIDS) (Table 12–1)

- Sudden death of an infant <12 mo that is unexplained after postmortem examination, investigation of the death scene, and review of the infant's case history
- Leading cause of death between 1 mo and 1 yr of age
- Incidence: two deaths/1000 live births
- Etiology
  - Many theories, no consensus
  - Agreement that there is no one single causative factor
  - Theories in review include
    - Brain stem abnormality affecting neurologic control of cardiorespiratory center
    - Prone position sleeping affecting oropharyngeal patency
    - Small airway occlusion
    - Cardiovascular abnormalities, especially electrical conduction abnormalities
    - Defects of metabolism
    - Infection

- Abnormal sleep and arousal states

ED treatment
- BLS and PALS resuscitation efforts
  - Initiated prehospital, in the ED, or not at all (per protocols)
- Obtain history
  - How the infant was found
  - Prehospital efforts
  - Past medical history
  - Prenatal and birth history

Table 12–1. Epidemiology of SIDS

Epidemiologic Factors	Occurrence
Incidence	1.4:1000 live births
Peak age	2–4 mo; 95% occur by 6 mo
Sex	Higher percentage of boys affected
Time of death	During sleep (vast majority)
Time of year	Increased incidence in winter
Race	Greater incidence in Native Americans and African-Americans
Socioeconomic factors	Increased occurrence in lower socioeconomic class
Birth	Higher incidence associated with prematurity, low birth weight, multiple births, low Apgar scores, central nervous system disturbances, respiratory disorders (e.g., BPD), increasing birth order (not the first born), recent history of illness
Sleep habits	Prone position, use of polystyrene-filled cushions, overheating
Feeding habits	Lower incidence in breast-fed infants
Siblings	May have greater incidence
Maternal factors	Young age, cigarette smoking (especially during pregnancy, substance abuse)

Modified from Wong D: Whaley and Wong's Nursing Care of Infants and Children, 5th ed. St. Louis, Mosby–Year Book, 1995.

SIDS support group _____

Medical examiner _____

Other _____

_____

_____

Figure 12–1. Form for providing SIDS information.

- Focus on the family following infant's death
  - Allow the family to say goodbye prior to discontinuation of resuscitation, if possible
  - Allow parents to hold the infant; don't rush them
  - Provide mementos, such as a lock of hair, footprints, or handprints
  - Provide delactation instructions for the nursing mother
  - Explain the diagnosis of SIDS to parents; answer their questions
  - Provide written SIDS materials and phone numbers of support groups, SIDS resources, and medical examiner's office (Fig. 12–1)

ASTHMA

- Chronic inflammatory lung disease
- Reactive airway disease (RAD)
- Prevalence rate increased 75% from 1980–1994 for all ages
  - 160% increase in ages 0–4 yr
  - 74% increase in ages 5–14 yr
- Characterized by
  - Airway hyperresponsiveness
  - Airway inflammation
  - Airway obstruction
- Airways are hyperresponsive to a variety of triggers
  - Allergens

- Environmental irritants
- Cold air
- Respiratory infections
- Exercise
- Triggers stimulate the release of inflammatory mediators
  - Resulting in airway obstruction by
    - Inflammation—edema and increased mucus (mucous plugging)
    - Smooth muscle contraction—bronchoconstriction
- Hypoxia results from mismatch of ventilation and perfusion

Signs and symptoms
- Dependent on severity of exacerbation
- Increased respiratory effort
  - Tachypnea (normal to >50% increase over baseline)
  - Use of accessory muscles
  - Retractions
  - Nasal flaring
  - Grunting respirations
- Other signs/symptoms
  - Complaints of chest discomfort or "heart hurting"
  - Difficulty drinking a bottle, shortness of breath, exercise intolerance
  - Softer and shorter cry
  - Speaks only in phrases, short sentences in child old enough to talk in sentences
  - Normal to pale or dusky skin color
  - "Tight" cough
  - Breath sounds
    - Prolonged expiratory phase
    - End-expiratory wheezes
    - Diffuse expiratory wheezes
    - Inspiratory and expiratory wheezes
    - "Silent chest"—minimal air exchange, if any, auscultated
  - Hypocapnia initially from hyperventilation,

followed by hypercapnia from continued obstruction
- Identification of infants and children at high risk for life-threatening exacerbations
  - Identify at triage
    - Asthma history includes
      - Prior intubation or intensive care unit (ICU) admission
      - Two or more hospitalizations within the past year
      - Three or more ED visits within the past year
      - ED or inpatient admission within the past month
      - Concomitant use of oral corticosteroids
      - Use of two or more canisters of short-acting bronchodilators per month
      - Comorbidity
    - "Silent chest"
    - Cyanosis
    - Decreased level of consciousness (LOC)
- Diagnostic studies
  - Pulse oximetry—at triage and prn
  - Peak expiratory flow rate (PEFR)
    - Objective assessment of airflow obstruction
    - For all children ≥5 yr
    - Initial PEFR at triage
    - Pre- and postbronchodilator PEFR measurements
    - Document on ED record
    - Determine predicted PEFR based on age and height
    - Ascertain patient's "personal best" PEFR if known
      - Use personal best PEFR for ED interventions and evaluations
  - CXR only for
    - First wheezing episode
    - Unilateral wheezing, suspected foreign body, pneumothorax, pneumonia

- Suspected infectious process, in presence of fever
- Severe exacerbation, nonresponsive to treatment
- Typical findings include hyperinflation, increased bronchial markings, and possibly atelectasis
- ABGs
  - Obtained to determine respiratory failure (hypercapnia) and evaluate need for additional interventions

ED treatment
- Inhaled beta$_2$-agonists (albuterol), given repetitively
  - First-line treatment
  - Most often via nebulization; may be given by metered dose inhaler (MDI) with spacer and observed correct technique
  - Use mask to administer nebulized medications to children <5 yr
  - Bronchodilator relaxes smooth muscle in airways
  - Onset of action is within 5 min
  - 0.15 mg/kg/dose up to 5 mg (minimum dose: 1.25 mg) every 20 min or continuous nebulization with 0.5 mg/kg/hr (maximum, 15 mg) via nebulizer
  - MDI—may give two puffs every 5 min up to 12 puffs, then four puffs every hour
- Systemic corticosteroids (prednisone, prednisolone)
  - Anti-inflammatory, moderate to severe exacerbations
  - Speeds resolution of obstruction
  - Reduces rate of relapse
  - Oral preparation has similar effectiveness as parenteral
  - Bad taste
    - Children often vomit after taking; repeat dose if emesis is immediately after administration

- Parenteral corticosteroids may be necessary
- Crushed prednisone tablet in a small amount (<3 mL) of juice may be more tolerable than liquid preparations
- 1–2 mg/kg initially given after two beta$_2$-agonists in the ED
- Onset of action in 3 hr, peak effectiveness 6–12 hr
- Discharged home with 1–2 mg/kg/day
  - No need to taper dose if given in "short burst" for 3–5 days
- Admitted child may receive 1–2 mg/kg q 6 hr
- Supplemental oxygen prn to maintain pulse oximetry at ≥95%
  - Don't "fight" with the child; oxygen demands will be driven higher
  - Blow-by oxygen as indicated for reluctant child
- Anticholinergics (ipratropium bromide)
  - Decrease vagal tone to airways
  - May be tried in children with poor response to initial therapy
  - 0.025% nebulizer solution, 0.025–0.05 mg/kg (maximum, 5 mg) every 6 hr
  - May be mixed in nebulizer with albuterol
  - If using a face mask with nebulizer, avoid leakage over nose/face, or blurred vision with or without eye pain may occur
- Status asthmaticus
  - Aggressive therapies include
    - Continuous nebulized albuterol
    - Systemic corticosteroids
    - Parenteral administration of beta$_2$-agonist
      - Epinephrine 1:1000 (1 mg/1 mL)
      - SQ: 0.01 mg/kg/dose (maximum, 0.3 mg)
      - Administer every 20 min × two doses
      - Greater risk of cardiotoxicity, especially in the hypoxic child
    - Continuous parenteral infusions of

- Terbutaline (beta$_2$-agonist)
  - Load with 10 μg or 0.01 mg/kg over 10 min
  - Continuous infusion of 0.1–4 μg/kg/min (maximum, 6 μg/kg/min)
  - Neb: 0.1–0.3 mg/kg/dose (maximum, 3 mg/dose) with 2.5 mL saline
  - SQ: 0.01 mg/kg/dose (maximum, 3 mg/dose) may repeat every 20 min up to three times
- Magnesium sulfate (controversial)
  - Direct smooth muscle relaxation
  - Involved in stabilization of mast cell membrane
  - 40 mg/kg over 20 min
  - Cardiorespiratory monitoring required
    - Observe for bradycardia, hypotension, hyporeflexia
- Ketamine
  - 1.0–2.5 mg/kg/hr by infusion
  - Relaxes bronchial smooth muscle
  - May increase catecholamine levels; observe for arrhythmias when using other beta-agonists
- Heliox
  - 80:20 mixture (helium:oxygen)
  - May be administered via mask
  - Ability to "go around" bronchoconstriction
  - Results seen within minutes
    - Lower airway pressures
    - Lower Pa$_{CO_2}$
- For the child in respiratory failure
  - Noninvasive positive pressure ventilation—BiPap, continuous positive airway pressure (CPAP)
  - Endotracheal intubation
    - For clinical deterioration
      - Fatigue
      - Altered mental status
    - "Permissive hypercapnia" or "con-

trolled hypoventilation" will minimize high airway pressures and barotrauma
  - Useful with inhalation and IV anesthetic agents
  - Fiberoptic bronchoscopy and lavage with acetylcysteine
    - Assist with removal of mucous plugs
  - Extracorporeal membrane oxygenation and carbon dioxide (CO_2) removal
- Disposition
  - Discharge to home
    - PEFR >70% predicted or personal best, minimal symptoms
    - Observe in ED at least 60 min after last bronchodilator
    - Continue systemic corticosteroids, if given, 3–10 days
    - Ensure follow-up with physician in 3–5 days
    - Caregiver instructions
      - Early warning signs of an asthma exacerbation
      - Signs of increased respiratory effort
      - When to call the physician/bring the child back to the ED
      - Medications
      - Correct medication administration techniques
      - Asthma diary/home monitoring
      - When and how often to use "quick reliever" medication
        - Beta$_2$-agonists
      - Triggers and environmental controls
  - Admit to hospital
  - Admit or transfer to pediatric ICU

BRONCHIOLITIS

- Lower respiratory tract viral illness
- Incidence
  - Most common 2–12 mo of age (rare after 2 yr)

- Most frequently seen in winter months and early spring
- High risk for severe disease
  - Prematurity, less than 34 wk gestational age
  - Less than 3 mo of age
  - Compromised cardiac, pulmonary, immune systems
    - Especially bronchopulmonary dysplasia (BPD)
    - Associated dehydration
- May be associated with
  - Crowded living conditions
  - Passive cigarette smoke exposure
  - Low socioeconomic status
- Transmission
  - Direct contact with respiratory secretions
  - Incubation of 5–8 days after exposure
- Etiologic agents
  - Most frequent is respiratory syncytial virus (RSV)
    - 50% of admissions for bronchiolitis
  - Others: adenoviruses, parainfluenza, rhinovirus, influenza
- Characterized by airway obstruction, especially on exhalation
  - Virus causes bronchiolar mucosal swelling
  - Lumens of bronchioles are filled with exudate and mucus
  - Air trapping and hyperinflation
    - Increased functional residual capacity
    - Diminished breath sounds
    - Apneic spells
- Diagnostic studies
  - Based on clinical findings
  - CXR
    - Hyperinflation
    - May also see interstitial infiltrates, atelectasis
  - CBC, although not usually helpful
  - Nasal secretions for RSV antigen

- Obtain via nasal washing or nasal swab
  - Nasal wash
    - Withdraw 2 mL saline from a vial using a butterfly-type needle
    - Cut off the needle, leaving the small tubing intact to the syringe with the saline
    - Insert the tubing into the child's nostril and instill the saline, followed by aspiration of the saline with nasal secretions
    - Place specimen in viral transport medium
- Rapid immunofluorescent antibody (IFA)
- Enzyme-linked immunosorbent assay (ELISA)
- Viral cultures
  - *Not* the test of choice; may take several days to get results

ED treatment
- Supportive care
- Humidity
- Contact isolation
  - Strict hand-washing
  - Placement in a private room if available
  - Viral shedding 3–8 days, may be as long as 4 wk
- Supplemental oxygen if oxygen saturation <95%
- Hydration
  - Consider IV hydration if tachypnea is severe
- Consider hospitalization for children with oxygen saturation <95% and severe distress
- Medications
  - Aerosolized bronchodilators—may be useful, although response varies
  - Corticosteroids—not medically proven to be beneficial
  - Antibiotics and cough suppressants—not proven to be beneficial

- Ribavirin
  - Antiviral agent
  - Not recommended for use in the ED
  - Communicate anticipated use in nursing report to inpatient unit
  - The only specific therapy for use with RSV
  - Potential toxic effects to health-care workers involved in care of child receiving ribavirin
    - Teratogenic effects in the laboratory only; none noted in actual clinical cases
- When used, follow recommendations of the American Academy of Pediatrics, Committee on Infectious Diseases, Committee on Fetus and Newborn Policy Statement. Respiratory Syncytial Virus Immune Globulin Intravenous: Indications for Use (RE9718). Volume 99, Number 4, 1997, pp 645–650.

BRONCHOPULMONARY DYSPLASIA (BPD)

- Chronic pulmonary disease
- Iatrogenic disease often associated with
  - High oxygen concentrations
  - Use of positive pressure ventilation
  - Endotracheal intubation
  - Fluid overload
  - Patent ductus arteriosus
- Infants most at risk
  - Premature infants more susceptible to respiratory distress syndrome, which may require therapies as listed previously
  - Meconium aspiration
  - Persistent pulmonary hypertension
  - Cyanotic heart disease
- Improved survival of extremely premature and low–birth-weight infants
  - Increased incidence overall of BPD
  - Decreased incidence of BPD in >30 wk gestation

- Widespread use of surfactant, high-frequency ventilation, use of steroids
- History of BPD is an important component of nursing history in high-risk infants who present to the ED
- Increased susceptibility to pulmonary infections
- BPD mortality largely due to pulmonary infections
- May be associated with growth and developmental delays
- Baseline CXR
  - Scattered atelectasis, patchy areas of hyperinflation

ED treatment
- Dependent on severity of presentation
- Oxygen to maintain oxygen saturation between 92–95%
  - Avoid hypoxia and hyperoxia
- Bronchodilators
- Diuretics
  - Maintain intake and output (I&O)
    - Assess for dehydration/pulmonary edema
- Discharge instructions dependent on presenting complaint and parental knowledge base

CROUP SYNDROMES (Table 12–2)

- Upper airway conditions that have varying degrees of obstruction
- Characterized by hoarseness and inspiratory stridor
- Include
  - Acute epiglottitis
  - Acute laryngotracheobronchitis (LTB)
  - Acute spasmodic laryngitis
  - Acute tracheitis

Table 12-2. Croup Syndromes

	Acute Epiglottitis	Acute LTB	Acute Spasmodic Laryngitis	Acute Tracheitis
Age group	1–8 yr	3 mo–8 yr	3 mo–3 yr	1 mo–6 yr
Etiologic agent	Bacterial—usually *H. influenzae*	Viral	Viral with allergic component	Bacterial—usually *Staphylococcus aureus*
Onset	Rapidly progressive	Slowly progressive	Sudden; at night	Moderately progressive
Major symptoms	Dysphagia Stridor aggravated when supine Drooling High fever Toxic appearance Rapid pulse and respirations	URI Stridor Brassy cough Hoarseness Dyspnea Restlessness Low-grade fever Irritability Nontoxic appearance	URI Croupy cough Stridor Hoarseness Dyspnea Restlessness Symptoms waken child Symptoms disappear during day Tends to recur	URI Croupy cough Stridor Purulent secretions High fever No response to LTB therapy
Treatment	Antibiotics Airway protection	Humidity Racemic epinephrine	Humidity	Antibiotics

URI, upper respiratory infection.
From Wong D: Whaley and Wong's Nursing Care of Infants and Children, 5th ed. St. Louis, Mosby–Year Book, 1995.

Acute epiglottitis

- Life-threatening
- Declining incidence since *Haemophilus influenzae* type B conjugate vaccine (Hib) became available
- Cardinal signs
  - Absence of spontaneous cough
  - Presence of drooling
  - Agitation
- ED treatment
  - Delay invasive diagnostic testing until airway is secured
  - Ensure that endotracheal intubation and cricothyroidotomy equipment is at bedside
    - Preferred location is in controlled operating room
  - Skilled personnel to accompany patient for all examinations
  - Diagnosis is usually made on history and examination
    - If unclear, may obtain a portable lateral neck x-ray
      - Read for presence of swollen epiglottis, "thumbprint"
        - Only seen in 50% of children
  - Antibiotics given IV ASAP after airway is secured
    - Ceftriaxone, cefotaxime, or cefuroxime
  - Corticosteroids may be helpful to reduce edema in the first 24 hr

Acute LTB

- Most common cause of upper airway obstruction in children
- Especially in fall and winter
- Transmitted via direct contact with respiratory secretions
- Mild (stage I) to severe (stage IV)
- Mild LTB
  - No stridor at rest
  - Usually managed at home

- Encourage oral fluids
- For symptoms, instruct parents to take child outside for 5 min and evaluate response
  - If not better, go to or return to the ED
- Severe LTB
  - Produces negative intrapleural pressure
  - May result in pulmonary edema
  - Severe inflammation responsible for ventilation-perfusion mismatch
    - Hypoxia, hypercarbia
  - ED treatment
    - Diagnosis based on history and examination
    - If unclear, x-rays
      - Lateral neck, read for presence of subglottic narrowing
      - Anteroposterior chest, read for subglottic "steeple" sign
        - Only seen in 40–50% of children
    - Administration of cool, humidified air
    - Supplemental oxygen if saturation <95%
    - Racemic epinephrine
      - Administered via nebulization
      - Produces vasoconstriction, reduces swelling
      - 2.25% solution, dosing
        - 0.05 mL/kg/dose (maximum, 0.5 mL) with 3 mL saline
      - Effect seen within 30 min
      - Duration 2 hr
      - May see return of severe symptoms as racemic epinephrine wears off
      - Observe all children in ED for 3–4 hr after administration of racemic epinephrine
    - Corticosteroids may be helpful to reduce edema in the first 24 hr

Acute Spasmodic Laryngitis

- Acute spasmodic croup, midnight croup, twilight croup

- Paroxysmal attacks of laryngeal obstruction occurring mostly at night
- May follow exposure to a precipitating factor
- Usually managed at home
- Severe cases treated as for LTB

Acute Tracheitis

- Severe cases may result in respiratory arrest
- Similar in presentation to LTB
- No response to LTB interventions
- Pseudomembranes may form over tracheal and laryngeal mucosa
  - May see as irregular tracheal margins on CXR
- Thick, purulent tracheal secretions
  - Produce respiratory distress
  - May require endotracheal intubation with frequent suctioning
- ED treatment
  - Early recognition with prompt administration of antibiotics
    - Broad-spectrum antibiotics

CYSTIC FIBROSIS (CF)

- Exocrine (mucus-producing) gland dysfunction
- Multisystem involvement
  - Respiratory, digestive, integumentary, and reproductive
- Characterized by
  - Increased viscosity of mucus
  - Elevation of sweat electrolytes
  - Changes in saliva
  - Autonomic nervous system dysfunction
- Suspected or rule out CF
  - Early diagnosis will enhance quality of life, though rarely diagnosed in the ED
  - Most common organic cause of failure to thrive
  - Diagnostic studies

- Sweat test—result indicating positive chlorides >60 mEq/L is definitive
- 72-hr fecal fat determination
- Liver enzymes—serum glutamic-oxaloacetic transaminase, serum glutamate pyruvate transaminase
- Fasting blood sugar
- CXR
- Sputum culture
- Pulmonary function testing

Signs and symptoms
- Clinical manifestations responsible for ED visit primarily respiratory
- Increased viscosity of mucus
  - Obstruction of bronchioles, both large and small airways
  - Stagnant mucus promotes growth of bacteria
    - *Staphylococcus aureus, Haemophilus influenzae, Streptococcus pneumoniae*, and *Pseudomonas aeruginosa* (seen later in disease)
  - Chronic infections cause damage to lung tissue
  - Fibrosis and scarring may result in ineffective gas exchange
    - Hypoxia, hypercapnia, and acidosis
    - Severe progression results in
      - Pulmonary hypertension, cor pulmonale, respiratory failure, death
    - Pneumothorax may result from ruptured bullae
    - Hemoptysis may result from erosion of bronchial wall into artery

ED treatment
- Oxygenation
  - Supplemental oxygenation may be necessary to maintain saturation >92%
  - Caution, many children with CF have chronic CO_2 retention
- Removal of mucopurulent secretions

- Chest physical therapy
- Aerosolized bronchodilators followed by chest physiotherapy
- Administration of antibiotics
- Obtain sputum culture
- CXR often obtained
- May require higher doses due to rapid metabolism of antibiotics by CF patients
- Many children with CF have venous access devices
- May discharge to home with IV antibiotics with established home-care nursing, if case not severe
- May also require systemic steroids
- Frequent assessments
  - Increasing respiratory effort or fatigue
  - Pulse oximetry
  - Pulmonary function tests/spirometry/peak flow measurements
  - Observe for development of pneumothorax
  - Hemoptysis
    - Blood-streaked sputum is common in children >10 yr old
    - Hemoptysis >300 mL in 24 hr indicates an emergent condition
    - Bed rest, cough suppressants, antibiotics
    - Prepare for bronchoscopy/surgery
    - Administration of vitamin K
- Avoid initiation of mechanical ventilation when possible; weaning is difficult
- Discuss end-of-life decisions with family as appropriate

DROWNING AND NEAR-DROWNING

- Definitions
  - Drowning: death from asphyxia while submerged, regardless of whether fluid has entered the lungs
    - Near-drowning: survival of at least 24 hr after submersion

- Drowning without aspiration—"dry drowning"
  - Death from respiratory obstruction and asphyxia while submerged, usually as a result of prolonged laryngospasm
  - 10% of drownings
- Drowning with aspiration—"wet drowning"
  - Death from combined effects of asphyxia and changes due to fluid aspiration while submerged
  - Initial aspiration causes laryngospasm and vomiting, glottis relaxes, lungs fill with fluid
- Near-drowning without aspiration and with aspiration may also occur
- Secondary drowning
  - Pulmonary edema not due to immediate drowning, but by later increases in capillary permeability
  - Occurs 24–72 hr after submersion
- Drowning
  - Most frequent in children <4 yr and >15 yr
    - Pulmonary changes that occur are caused by
      - Length of submersion
      - Physiologic response of victim
        - Younger children tolerate longer periods of submersion
        - Drowning reflex (a.k.a. diving reflex)
          - Neurologic response triggered by immersion of face in cold water
          - Blood is shunted away from periphery; blood delivered to essential organs only
          - Profound bradycardia
      - Degree of development of hypothermia
- Near-drowning
  - Results in
    - Hypoxia and asphyxiation
    - Aspiration resulting in
      - Pulmonary edema

- Atelectasis
- Pneumonitis
- Hypothermia
- Salt water versus fresh water
  - No significant clinical difference in outcomes
  - Salt water
    - Hypertonic fluid drawn into alveoli dilutes surfactant
    - Hypovolemia, hemoconcentration
    - Increased serum electrolytes
  - Fresh water
    - Fluid drawn out of alveoli into intravascular space
    - Surfactant is denatured, alveoli collapse and pulmonary shunting occurs
    - Hypervolemia, hemodilution
    - Decreased serum electrolytes

ED treatment
- Airway, breathing, and circulation (ABCs)
- Priority: oxygenation and ventilation
  - Continuous pulse oximetry, end-tidal CO_2 measurements
  - Assist respirations as needed, 100% FIO_2
  - Mechanical ventilation for respiratory failure, metabolic acidosis, cerebral edema
    - Positive end-expiratory pressure (PEEP)/CPAP if evidence of progressive pulmonary edema
  - Guide resuscitation by ABGs
  - Nebulized beta$_2$-agonists for bronchospasm
  - Obtain core rectal or esophageal temperature
    - Initiate measures to achieve and maintain normothermia
  - CBC, electrolytes, serum osmolarity, blood urea nitrogen, creatinine, alcohol, drug screens
  - Assess for signs of associated trauma, especially head and neck trauma

- CXR
  - Variable findings: scattered infiltrates to pulmonary edema
  - Check endotracheal tube placement
- Nasogastric tube insertion
- Urinary catheter insertion with accurate I&O
- Computed axial tomography scan
- Monitor neurologic status, observe for signs of increased intracranial pressure (ICP)
  - ICP monitoring where available
  - Elevate head of bed 30° if stable
  - Mannitol (0.5 g/kg/dose over 30 min) for increased ICP
  - Paralysis and sedation for the intubated child may be necessary
  - Control hypoxic seizures with oxygenation, ventilation, and
    - Diazepam 0.2–0.3 mg/kg/dose *or*
    - Lorazepam 0.05–0.15 mg/kg/dose over 1–3 min
  - Lasix (1–3 mg/kg/dose) for diuresis
  - Hospitalized 12–24 hr for observation
  - Observe for aspiration pneumonia 48–72 hr after submersion
- Prognosis
  - Best: submersion in non-icy water <10 min; responsive at the scene
    - Young age, core temperature >35°C
    - No clinical signs of aspiration
  - Worst: submerged >10 min; no response to advanced life support after 25 min
    - <3 yr old
    - Initial delay in resuscitation measures at the scene
    - Presence of seizures, posturing, fixed and dilated pupils, coma
    - Arterial pH <7.10
- Prevention

- Stress adequate supervision around any body of water
- Encourage safety measures around pools
  - Fences, alarms, pool covers
    - Advocate water safety and swimming/ survival instruction
    - Encourage parents with pools to learn CPR

PERTUSSIS (WHOOPING COUGH)
(Tables 12–3, 12–4)

- Suspect in poorly immunized children
- Causative agent: *Bordetella pertussis*, a gram-negative rod
- Peak incidence, late summer and early fall
- Children usually <4 yr
- Higher morbidity and mortality in children <1 yr
- Inflammatory response of the respiratory tract
  - Bronchiolar congestion

Table 12–3. Three Stages of Pertussis

Stage	Duration	Symptoms
Catarrhal	1–2 wk	Minor upper respiratory infection symptoms, conjunctivitis
Paroxysmal	2–4 wk	Paroxysms of severe coughing and inspiratory "whoop"; may have 40 episodes a day; frequently worse at night; often associated with posttussive emesis (young infants may not have characteristic "whoop"; may have periods of apnea)
Convalescent	1–4 wk	Gradual improvement, cough may last 6 mo

Table 12–4. Complications Associated With Pertussis

Complication	Etiology
Subcutaneous emphysema, ruptured diaphragm, epistaxis, subconjunctival hemorrhages	Forceful coughing
Atelectasis	Mucous plugging
Pneumonia	Secondary infection
Seizures, encephalopathy	Toxin-mediated effects
Alkalosis	Persistent vomiting

- Obstruction
- Necrosis
- Transmission
  - Direct contact with respiratory secretions
  - Droplet spread
  - Indirect contact with contaminated objects
  - Most communicable during catarrhal stage, before paroxysms of coughing begin
  - Incubation usually 7–10 days
- Signs and symptoms
  - More severe symptoms in younger infants
- Diagnostic studies
  - Nasopharyngeal (NP) culture, NP swab
  - WBC—elevated with lymphocytosis
  - CXR may show infiltrates, "shaggy" heart border

ED treatment
- Supplemental humidified oxygen to maintain Spo_2 ≥95%
- Avoid use of mist—it may trigger paroxysm of coughing
- Suction thick secretions prn—avoid deep suctioning
- Monitor heart rhythm and rate, hydration, and respiratory status

- Maintain respiratory isolation in ED and after admission, usually until 5th day of antibiotics
- IV access
- Antibiotic therapy
  - Best if given early in catarrhal stage
  - Erythromycin 20–30 mg/kg/24 hr
  - Administered every 6 hr for 14 days
  - Treat exposed individuals with antibiotics for 10 days
- Bedside glucose
- ABGs as needed for severe distress
- Nebulized albuterol
- Systemic corticosteroids
- Avoid the use of cough suppressants
- Disposition
  - Inpatient admission
    - <6 mo old
    - Dehydrated
    - Presence of complications (see Table 12–4)
  - Discharge home
    - Discharge instructions include
      - Communicability, hydration, medication administration, environmental trigger controls
      - Demonstrate gentle nasal suctioning in infants
  - Prevention
    - Adequate immunization of infants and children

PNEUMONIA (Table 12–5)

- Inflammation, most frequently with infection of pulmonary parenchyma
- Occurs as primary illness or secondary to another illness, injury, aspiration
- Types include viral, bacterial, fungal, parasitic, or other atypical organisms
  - Viral and bacterial most common
  - Viral occurs more frequently
  - Atypical organisms include *Chlamydia trachomatis* and *Mycobacterium tuberculosis*

Table 12–5. Types of Pneumonia With Characteristic Features

	Viral	Bacterial	Mycoplasmal
Causative agent	RSV, parainfluenza, influenza, adenovirus, rhinovirus	*Streptococcus pneumoniae, Staphylococcus aureus, Haemophilus influenzae* (seen much less since use of Hib vaccine)	*Mycoplasma pneumoniae*
Age	All ages; most common in children <5 yr	All ages	Most common in children >5 yr
Onset	Gradual	Rapid	Gradual
Fever	Moderate	High, often with chills	Low
Cough	Dry	Productive (child often swallows sputum, resulting in nausea and vomiting)	Dry, hacking cough, especially at night; may become productive
Breath sounds	Few crackles, few wheezes	Decreased breath sounds, crackles, rhonchi	Fine crackles, rare wheezes
Other signs or symptoms	Severity of symptoms vary; myalgias common CXR: diffuse or patchy infiltrates WBCs normal	Pleuritic pain, anorexia CXR: diffuse or patchy infiltrates WBCs increased, often >15,000 cells/mm^3 and increased bands	Headache, pharyngitis, malaise, anorexia CXR: May show areas of consolidation WBCs normal
Specific ED treatment	Supportive care; child is susceptible to a secondary bacterial infection	Supportive care and antibiotics Young child: PO—amoxicillin-clavulanate (Augmentin); parenteral—ampicillin, ceftriaxone, or nafcillin School-age child: PO—erythromycin; parenteral—ampicillin, ceftriaxone, or nafcillin	Supportive care and antibiotics: erythromycin

- *C. trachomatis* most common in neonates
  - Newborns acquire infection from mothers during the birth process
  - Usually seen in infants between 1 and 3 mo old
  - Characterized by persistent staccato cough, tachypnea, and conjunctivitis
  - Antibiotics of choice are erythromycin or sulfa drugs
- Children with chronic disease and congenital defects are more susceptible
- Overcrowded conditions predispose children to pneumonia
- Infants from homes with smokers have twice the risk of developing pneumonia and bronchitis
- ED supportive care and monitoring for the child with pneumonia
  - Thorough and ongoing respiratory assessments
    - Respiratory rate and quality of respirations
    - Use of accessory muscles, retractions, nasal flaring
    - Color
    - Breath sounds
    - LOC, age-appropriate behavior, restlessness
  - Supplemental humidified oxygen to maintain SpO_2 at $\geq$95%
  - Medication administration
    - Antibiotics
    - Antipyretics
    - Bronchodilators if bronchospasm is present
    - Expectorants of questionable value
    - Antitussives with codeine are reserved for child who is having difficulty sleeping/resting due to persistent cough
  - Maintain hydration
    - Oral fluids as tolerated
    - IV fluids

- Consider insensible losses through fever, tachypnea
- Allow child to adopt position of comfort
- Encourage family to participate in supportive care for child
- Suction as needed
- Chest physiotherapy and postural drainage as needed
- Disposition
  - Most children with pneumonia are treated and released from the ED
  - Hospitalization may be necessary for
    - Significant toxicity
      - Apnea, cyanosis, fatigue
    - Presence of respiratory failure
    - Ill-appearing infants <3 mo of age
    - Children with chronic illness or congenital defect placing them at high risk for complications
    - Presence of pleural effusions
    - Requirement for supplemental oxygen
- Prevention
  - Encourage parents to adopt a no smoking policy in their home
  - Encourage children at risk to obtain influenza and pneumococcal vaccines
  - Demonstrate proper hand-washing techniques

RESPIRATORY FAILURE (Table 12–6)

- A common cause of cardiopulmonary arrest in children
- Signs are often subtle
- Children are able to compensate for illness or injury for a long time
- Depletion of compensatory reserves results in cardiopulmonary arrest
- Few children who arrest survive; of those who do, many are left with neurologic deficits
- Respiratory failure

Table 12–6. Special Considerations of Respiratory Failure in Children

Children Have	Resulting In
Small, compliant airways	Easily obstructed due to mucus, edema
Increased airway resistance from smaller, obstructed airways	Increased work of breathing and oxygen consumption
Immature thoracic wall	Retractions; respiratory muscles are easily fatigued
High oxygen consumption rate	Rapid decompensation with unmet demands for oxygen or severely limited supply of oxygen

- A clinical condition
- Characterized by inadequate gas exchange
  - Retained CO_2
  - Hypoxemia
- Most commonly due to upper or lower obstructive lung disease
  - Other causes
    - Restrictive lung disease
    - Primary inefficient gas transfer
      - Respiratory center depression
      - Pulmonary diffusion defects

ED treatment
- Establish vascular access
- Establish monitoring
  - Pulse oximeter
  - Cardiorespiratory monitor
  - Noninvasive blood pressure
  - End-tidal CO_2 or capnography after intubation
- Suction as needed
- Insert gastric tube
- Provide comfort measures, pain control, sedation as indicated

- Establish normothermia (control oxygen consumption and CO_2 production)
- Identify underlying cause and treat appropriately
- Provide explanations, reassurance, and support for family members
  - Consider allowing family presence during emergent interventions

Selected Bibliography

Barkin RM, Rosen P: Emergency Pediatrics A Guide to Ambulatory Care, 4th ed. St. Louis, Mosby–Year Book, 1994.

Betz CL, Sowden LA: Mosby's Pediatric Nursing Reference, 3rd ed. St. Louis, Mosby–Year Book, 1996.

Broyles BE: Clinical Companion for Ashwill and Droske Nursing Care of Children: Principles and Practice. Philadelphia, W.B. Saunders, 1997.

Chameides L, Hazinski MF (eds): Textbook of Pediatric Advanced Life Support. Dallas, American Heart Association, 1994.

Haley K, Baker P (eds): Instructor Manual Emergency Nursing Pediatric Nursing Course. Chicago, Emergency Nurses Association, 1993.

Soud TE, Rogers JS: Manual of Pediatric Emergency Nursing. St. Louis, Mosby–Year Book, 1998.

Wong DL: Whaley and Wong's Nursing Care of Infants and Children, 5th ed. St. Louis, Mosby–Year Book, 1995.

Chapter 13
Surface Trauma/Bites and Stings

SOFT-TISSUE INJURY

- Can affect
  - Skin (epidermis, dermis)
  - Subcutaneous adipose tissue
  - Veins, arteries, and nerves
  - Tendons
  - Muscle

Abrasion

- Epithelial layer is scraped away
- Partial-thickness denuding
- Ranges from small to large surface areas

Avulsion

- Full-thickness skin loss
- Section of skin is pulled away
- Wound edge approximation is prevented because of loss of skin
- Severe avulsions may require skin grafting

Contusion

- No break in the skin
- Extravasation of blood into the tissues
- Blunt trauma, crush, or wringer-type injuries
- Ecchymosis and swelling result in pain

SUBUNGUAL HEMATOMA

- A type of contusion
- Blood vessel(s) traumatized under a fingernail or toenail
- In cases of questionable fracture, get an x-ray before releasing a subungual hematoma
  - Release (if fractured) can result in an "open" fracture
    - In the presence of a fracture, antibiotics should be prescribed
    - Release is accomplished by use of a cautery needle through the nail with drainage of trapped blood/fluid

Laceration

- Open wound
- Cuts, slices through dermal layer or deeper
- Results from sharp cut, slice, or tear
- Varies in length and depth
- Can have a "flap"
- Repair >12 hr (if done at all) requires meticulous skin preparation, wound edge excision, and approximation of wound edges
  - Greater chance for infection after 6–8 hr
- Chin, scalp, extremities are common sites of lacerations on children

Puncture Wounds

- Skin layer penetrated by a sharp object
  - Nail
  - Tack
  - Toothpick
- High potential for infection
- Foreign body retention is a consideration

Foreign Body (FB)

- Embedded or retained in the skin, subcutaneous tissue, or muscle

- Broken needles, splinters (e.g., wood, bamboo)
- Pins, fish hooks
  - Rubber (e.g., from tennis shoes after stepping on a nail)
  - Cloth (driven into skin with the FB)
  - Graphite (from pencil)
- High potential for infection
- X-rays may be necessary to locate the FB
  - Puncture site is marked

Emergency Department (ED) Treatment for Surface Injury

- Airway, breathing, and circulation (ABCs)
- Assess color, movement, sensation, and pulses distal to the wound
- Consider local anesthesia if needed for thorough cleansing (Table 13–1)
- Thorough cleansing and, if necessary, débridement
  - Prevents tattooing of skin
- Hemostasis as indicated
  - Direct/indirect pressure
- Elevation of affected areas
- Wound closure as indicated
- Sterile dressings (ranges from adhesive bandages to bulky dressings)
- Antibiotics as indicated
- Instructions for wound recheck, home care, and suture removal
- Tetanus prophylaxis

Skin Closure Materials

Suture (Table 13–2)

- Absorbable Suture
  - Gut
    - Plain
    - Chromic

Table 13–1. Local Anesthetics

Drug	Administration Considerations
Topical Preparations	
TAC: Tetracaine 1%, adrenaline 1%, cocaine hydrochloride 4%	Ascertain allergy. TAC and XAP not for use on mucosal lesions or when adrenaline is contraindicated; great for young children to preanesthetize area prior to local infiltration before suturing.
XAP: Xylocaine 2%, adrenaline 1%, pontocaine 2%	Apply solution to cotton ball or swab and hold over the wound for 10–15 min. Topical lidocaine can be used for cold sores and
Topical lidocaine (Xylocaine) 2%, 4%	oral pain; not for application to large areas
Infiltrative Solutions	
Lidocaine (Xylocaine) 1%, 2%	Onset 5–15 min; duration 1–2 hr; infiltration is performed directly through wound margins using syringe with 25 to 27 gauge needle
Buffered lidocaine	Mixture of sodium bicarbonate and lidocaine in 1:10 ratio; shelf life is 1 wk; pH is neutralized to minimize injection discomfort
Lidocaine with epinephrine 1%, 2%	Use only in areas of good tissue perfusion; not for use on digits, ears, hands, feet, penis
Bupivacaine (Marcaine) 0.25%, 0.5%, 0.75%	Onset 10–30 min; duration 4–8 hr; also used for epidural and caudal anesthesia and peripheral nerve block

Table 13–2. Suture Sizes and Repair Sites (Examples)

Size	Skin Layer	Sites of Repair
3-0, 4-0	Fascia, muscle, subcutaneous tissue	Scalp, knee, elbow
5-0	Dermis	Fingers, hands
6-0	Dermis	Facial areas
7-0, 8-0	Skin, vessels, nerves	Microscopic repair of nailbed lacerations

- Vicryl
- Dexon
- Polydioxanone
- Nonabsorbable suture
  - Dacron
  - Nylon
  - Prolene
  - Ethibond
  - Wire
  - Silk

Staples

- Good for uncomplicated scalp lacerations
- Quick, easy to approximate a wound
- Removed with surgical staple remover

Tape Closures

- For wounds that approximate well
- Must keep dry and intact until edges start to peel (or 3–7 days)
- Must have parental/caregiver ability to keep dry

BITES

Human

- Common in children, especially toddlers and small children
- Considered a "dirty" wound
  - Multiple organisms in mouth, saliva, and on teeth
    - Closure is dependent on severity of the wound due to high risk for infection
- May have teeth marks, ecchymosis, swelling
- May require IV antibiotics if severe

Animal

- Reportable to local police or animal control
- Canine teeth can cause deep puncture wounds and/or tearing of skin
  - Closure is dependent on severity of the wound due to high risk for infection
- Rabies can be carried by
  - Raccoons
  - Bats
  - Squirrels
  - Skunks
  - Opossums
  - Cats
  - Dogs

RABIES POSTEXPOSURE TREATMENT

- Rabies immune globulin, Human (Hyperab, Imogam)
  - Dose for children
  - 20 units/kg IM (gluteal)
    - Infiltrate ½ the dose locally around the wound
    Give the remainder IM
- Given with Human Diploid Cell Cultures Rabies Vaccine (HDCV)
  - Rabies Virus Vaccine, HDCV (Immovax)

- Dose
  - 1 mL IM on days 1, 3, 7, 14, and 28
  - Given IM only
- RATS mnenomic
  - **R** = **R**abies vaccine
  - **A** = **A**ntibiotics
  - **T** = **T**etanus prophylaxis
  - **S** = **S**crub with lots of *S*oap

SNAKE BITES

- Important to know snakes common to your area
- Children, especially boys, will pick up or try to capture snakes

Types

- Pit viper
  - Rattlesnake
  - Cottonmouth
  - Copperhead
  - Water moccasin
- Elapids
  - Coral snake
    - How to tell a coral snake (poisonous) from similar-looking nonpoisonous snakes (refers to the colored bands on the snake):
      Red touch yellow
      Kill a fellow
      Red touch black
      Okay for Jack
  - Cobra
- Viperids
  - Puff adder
- Hydrophids
  - Sea snakes
- Colubrids
  - Boomslang

Venoms

- Cause tissue destruction
- Injected via snake fangs

- Manufactured in salivary glands, stored in the fangs
- Some venoms are cardiotoxic, neurotoxic, hemotoxic, or combination

ED Treatment

- Keep extremity in dependent position and immobilized
- Antivenom (polyvalent) if severe reaction
- Tetanus prophylaxis
- IV access
  - Treat symptoms of shock
  - IV antibiotics as needed

ARACHNID AND INSECT BITES AND STINGS

Spiders

- Black widow
  - Black body
  - Red hourglass on abdomen
  - Neurotoxic venom
  - Treat the symptoms, which may include shock
- Brown recluse
  - Light brown body
  - Dark brown fiddle shape on back
  - Local reactions
    - Edema
    - Bluish ring around the bite area
    - Bleb formation
- Systemic reactions
- Fever
- Nausea and/or vomiting
- Weakness
- Joint pain
- Petechiae
- Severe signs of shock, disseminated intravascular coagulation (DIC), cardiac arrest

ED TREATMENT

- ABCs
- Aggressive treatment
- IV access
  - Possible fluid resuscitation for shock
  - IV calcium (black widow)
- Antivenom if severe reaction
- Application of ice to affected area
- Wound débridement (brown recluse)
- Pain control

Stinging Insects

- Hymenoptera order
  - Bees (yellowjackets, honeybees), wasps, hornets, fire ants
- Allergic reactions can result in significant morbidity in children

SIGNS AND SYMPTOMS

- Reactions are immediate to delayed
- Anaphylaxis is most severe reaction
  - Urticaria
  - Flushing of skin
  - Angioedema
  - Cardiovascular collapse
    - Hypotension
  - Respiratory involvement
    - Edema of pharynx
    - Bronchospasm

ED TREATMENT

- ABCs
- IV access if systemic reaction
- Epinephrine 0.01 mL/kg of a 1:1000 solution (pediatric dose)
  - Maximum dose is 0.3 mL
- Vasopressor agents

- Glucocorticoids to prevent recurrent or prolonged symptoms
- Remove the stinger (if any)
  - Scrape with a credit card or stiff cardboard
  - Do not use forceps to grasp (may inject more toxin)
- Treat local reactions
  - Ice bag
  - Elevation
  - Antihistamines
- Many local residents treat fire ant bites with dilute ammonia applied topically to the affected area

Ticks

- Attach or burrow under the skin
- Flaccid paralysis can occur from neurotoxin

ROCKY MOUNTAIN SPOTTED FEVER

- Symptoms 2–5 days after tick bite
  - Fever
  - Chills
  - Headache
  - Photophobia
  - Muscle and joint pain
- Characteristic skin rash initially on ankles and wrists; spreads to trunk, palms of hands, and soles of feet

LYME DISEASE

- Endemic to Minnesota, Wisconsin, California, Texas, and Nevada
- More prominent in summer months
- Symptoms progress in stages after tick bite
  - Stage 1 symptoms appear in 3–32 days
    - Characteristic skin rash begins as small red spot and develops into a reddish circle resembling a "bull's eye"
    - Headache

- Fatigue
- Myalgia
- Stage 2 symptoms appear within 5 wk
  - Myocarditis
  - Atrioventricular node blocks
    - May require pacemaker insertion
  - Aseptic meningitis
  - Encephalitis
  - Bell's palsy of cranial nerve VII
- Stage 3 symptoms can develop within weeks to years
  - Intermittent arthritis resembling juvenile rheumatoid arthritis (JRA) (see Chapter 11)
    - Have negative rheumatoid factor and antinuclear antibody

ED TREATMENT

- ABCs
- Serologic testing
- Antibiotic therapy to prevent complications
- Must rule out JRA
- Treat systemic involvement

Selected Bibliography

Ashwill J, Droske S: Nursing Care of Children: Principles and Practice. Philadelphia, W.B. Saunders, 1997.

Behrman R, Kliegman R: Nelson Essentials of Pediatrics. Philadelphia, W.B. Saunders, 1998.

Budassi Sheehy S: Emergency Nursing Principles and Practice, 3rd ed. St. Louis, Mosby–Year Book, 1992.

Emergency Nurses Association: Emergency Nursing Core Curriculum, 4th ed. Philadelphia, W.B. Saunders, 1994.

Green N, Swiontkowski M: Skeletal Trauma in Children. Vol. 3. Philadelphia, W.B. Saunders, 1998.

Selfridge-Thomas J: Manual of Emergency Nursing. Philadelphia, W.B. Saunders, 1995.

Skidmore-Roth L: Nursing Drug Reference. St. Louis, Mosby–Year Book, 1993.

Sound T, Rogers J: Manual of Pediatric Emergency Nursing. St. Louis, Mosby–Year Book, 1998.

Subcommittee on Pharmacy and Therapeutics: The U of C Hospitals Formulary. Chicago, University of Chicago, 1995.

Tipsord-Klinkhammer B, Andreoni C: Quick Reference for Emergency Nursing. Philadelphia, W.B. Saunders, 1998.

Chapter 14
Toxicologic

- May be intentional or accidental
- Exposure may be by inhalation, dermal, ocular, ingestion, or parenteral routes
- Components of the history include
  - Type and amount of substance
  - Route
  - Time of exposure
  - Treatment given prior to arrival in the emergency department (ED)
- The most common items ingested by children are
  - Soaps and detergents
  - Plants
  - Medications and vitamins
  - Household products
- Therapy is directed toward airway, breathing, and circulation (ABCs), elimination of toxin, and prevention of further absorption (Table 14–1)

ACETAMINOPHEN POISONING

- Found in many over-the-counter (OTC) preparations
- May cause delayed hepatic toxicity
- Three phases of poisoning
  - Phase I: within first few hours
    - Vomiting
    - Malaise
    - Anorexia
    - Pallor
  - Phase II: next 48 hr
    - Typically asymptomatic
    - May have mild GI symptoms

Table 14–1. Toxic Syndromes

Syndrome	Manifestations	Common Causes
Narcotic	Central nervous system (CNS) depression, miosis, hypotension, hypoventilation	Narcotics, sedatives, diphenoxylate with atropine (Lomotil), propoxyphene, benzodiazepines, methaqualone, glutethimide, and pentazocine
Cholinergic	Salivation, urination, lacrimation, defecation, gastrointestinal cramping, emesis, miosis	Organophosphate and carbamate insecticides, physostigmine, neostigmine
Anticholinergic	Confusion, incoordination, hallucinations, delirium, dry skin and mucous membranes, tachycardia, mydriasis, fever, urinary retention, decreased bowel sounds	Belladonna alkaloids, certain mushrooms, antihistamines, tricyclic antidepressants, over-the-counter (OTC) sleep medications, scopolamine, jimsonweed
Sympathomimetic	CNS excitation, tachycardia, seizures, hypertension	OTC cough and cold preparations, (phenylpropanolamine), theophylline, caffeine, lysergic acid diethylamide, PCP, amphetamines

From Wruk K, Montanio C: Toxicological emergencies. *In* Emergency Nurses Association (ed): Emergency Nursing Core Curriculum, 4th ed. Philadelphia, W.B. Saunders, 1994.

- May have mild right upper quadrant (RUQ) tenderness
- Decreased urinary output
- Phase III: 3–5 days
  - Acute hepatic necrosis
  - Renal failure
  - Jaundice
  - RUQ pain
  - Hepatomegaly
  - Encephalopathy
  - Myocardiopathy

ED Treatment

- ABCs
- Gastric emptying by lavage
- Do not delay charcoal administration, regardless of whether N-acetylcysteine (NAC) is being considered
  - Charcoal does not significantly decrease effect of NAC
- Consider toxic: ingestion of >150 mg/kg (child)
- Antidote: NAC for toxic ingestion (Fig. 14–1)
  - Dosage = 140 mg/kg PO initial dose, then 70 mg/kg PO q 4 hr for 17 doses; dilute 10–20% solution to 5% with juice or soda to mask taste
  - NAC is most effective within 16 hr of acetaminophen ingestion
  - IV NAC may be considered for the patient with persistent vomiting not controlled by antiemetics (call Rocky Mountain Poison Center, 800-525-6115, for administration information)
- Monitor liver function tests

ACID AND ALKALI INGESTION

- Acids cause severe burns to the GI tract and coagulation necrosis

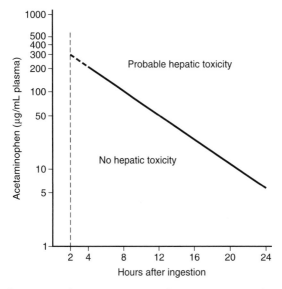

Figure 14–1. Semilogarithmic plot of plasma acetaminophen levels versus time. (From Rumak BH, Matthew H: Acetaminophen poisoning and toxicity. Pediatrics 55:871–876, 1975.)

- Alkalis may cause tissue necrosis within 1 sec of exposure
- Alkali esophageal burns
  - Phase I: 1–2 days (inflammatory phase); perforation may occur
  - Phase II: 24–48 hr after ingestion (necrotic phase); sloughing of tissue
  - Phase III: 2–6 wk after ingestion (constriction phase); narrowing of esophagus
- Coffee-ground emesis
- Dysphagia, drooling, chest discomfort
- Oral or pharyngeal burns
- Respiratory distress may develop because of soft tissue swelling of upper airway
- Esophageal perforation may result in mediastinitis and shock

ED Treatment

- ABCs
- Flush lips, mouth with copious amounts of water
- Dilute with milk (may use water if milk not available)
- For significant ingestion
  - Complete blood count (CBC), type and crossmatch, arterial blood gases (ABGs)
  - Cardiac monitor, pulse oximetry
  - Lateral neck, chest, abdominal x-rays
- Esophagoscopy is performed within 12–24 hr after alkali ingestion
- Do *not* induce vomiting; lavage or give charcoal
- Absence of oropharyngeal burns does not exclude esophageal injury
- Dilution of ingested material is contraindicated if perforation, shock, or respiratory distress is present
- Call the National Button & Battery Ingestion Hotline, 202-625-3333, in Washington, DC, for information on chemical content of batteries and clinical management recommendations

BARBITURATE POISONING

General Information

- CNS depressants
- Toxicity is enhanced by alcohol and depressants
- Includes
  - Phenobarbital (long acting)
  - Amobarbital, butabarbital (intermediate acting)
  - Pentobarbital, secobarbital (short acting)
  - Thiopental (ultra–short acting)

Signs and Symptoms

- Altered level of consciousness (LOC), coma
- Slurred speech

- Ataxia
- Hypotension
- Respiratory arrest
- Bullae over pressure points (barbiturate burns)
- Pupillary constriction
- Hyporeflexia
- Dysconjugate eye movements
- Hypothermia

ED Treatment

- ABCs
- Gastric lavage (emesis contraindicated due to possible rapid decrease in LOC)
- Administration of charcoal and cathartic (first dose)
  - Repeated doses of charcoal alone are recommended to enhance elimination and shorten the half-life of phenobarbital
- Alkalinization of urine or hemodialysis is only effective for phenobarbital

CARBON MONOXIDE (CO) POISONING

- Commonly affects more than one person (e.g., a whole family)
- Due to poor ventilation of stove, furnace, automobile exhaust, smoldering charcoal, canned heat, and wood fires
- A colorless, odorless gas
- Binds with hemoglobin at the expense of oxygen, resulting in tissue hypoxia

Signs and Symptoms

- Chronic exposure
  - Recurring headaches, dizziness, nausea that are severe on awakening and improve after leaving the home
- Acute exposure

- Headache
- Nausea and vomiting
- Loss of consciousness
- Decreased respiratory rate
- Decreased heart rate
- Seizures/twitching
- Hypotension
- Cherry red color of the blood and skin
- Elevated carboxyhemoglobin values
  - Normal values
    - Nonsmoker = <3%
    - Smoker = up to 12%
    - Newborn = up to 12%
  - Critical values
    - >20% = symptoms of dizziness, headache, disturbances in judgment
    - 30–40% = symptoms of tachycardia, hypercapnea, hypotension, confusion
    - 50–60% = coma
    - >60% = death

ED Treatment

- ABCs
- 100% oxygen via non-rebreather mask
- Monitor cardiac rhythm
- Obtain ABGs and carboxyhemoglobin level initially and 6–12 hr after treatment
- Hyperbaric oxygen may be required
  - Unconsciousness
  - Ischemic changes on electrocardiogram (EKG)
  - Carboxyhemoglobin levels >25%
- Household pets may be reported dead by prehospital care providers who transport a family with suspected CO poisoning to the ED

HEAVY METAL POISONING

- Heavy metals include arsenic, lead, mercury
  - Lead poisoning is a common and preventable pediatric health problem

- Sources include lead-based paint, dust, and soil
- Heavy metals deposit in the body and are excreted slowly

Signs and Symptoms

- CNS, lungs, liver, and kidneys are especially susceptible
- Signs and symptoms of common heavy metals poisoning
  - Arsenic
    - Garlicky breath
    - Profuse rice-like diarrhea
    - Polyneuropathy
    - Abnormal kidney, ureter, and bladder
    - Vomiting, abdominal pain
    - Dysrhythmias
    - Cutaneous abnormalities
  - Lead
    - Weakness, irritability, ataxia
    - Weight loss
    - Personality changes
    - Severe abdominal pain
    - Milky vomiting
    - Hypertension
    - Peripheral neuropathy
    - Coma, seizures
  - Mercury
    - Stomatitis
    - Colitis
    - Ataxia
    - Gingivitis
    - Nephrotic syndrome

ED Treatment

- ABCs
- Obtain blood specimen for levels of metal 1–2 hr post ingestion and repeat 2–4 hr later and prn during chelation therapy
- Monitor urine output and urine concentration of metal

- CBC, blood urea nitrogen, creatinine, electrolytes, liver function, and renal function tests
- Begin 24-hr urine collection
- Specific for lead
  - Erythrocyte protoporphyrin level
  - Urine lead levels
  - X-ray of abdomen, knees, wrists (lead is radiopaque and deposits may be seen at these sites)
- See specific therapy (Table 14–2)

IRON TOXICITY

- Ingestion is most common route
- Iron tablets are often mistaken for candy by children

Clinical Effects

- GI symptoms (30 min–6 hr after ingestion)
  - Nausea
  - Vomiting/hematemesis
  - Diarrhea
  - Abdominal pain
- Latent period (6–24 hr after ingestion)
- Systemic symptoms (4–40 hr after ingestion)
  - Acidosis
  - Cyanosis
  - Fever
  - Shock
- Liver and renal failure (2–4 days after ingestion)
- Late complications (2–8 wk after ingestion)
  - GI obstruction and scarring
- Iron toxicity can be seen in children with sickle cell disease who are being treated with long-term transfusion therapy
  - May exhibit iron deposits in organs

ED Treatment

- ABCs
- Serum iron levels, coagulation studies, stool

Table 14–2. Chelation and Metal Specific Therapies

Metal	Antidote	Dosage
Arsenic, mercury, gold	British antilewisite (BAL) (dimercaprol)	5 mg/kg IM as soon as possible
Lead	Edetate calcium (calcium disodium versenate)	1500 mg/m²/day × 5 days; divided q 6 hr or given by continuous infusion
	BAL	500 mg/m²/day IM divided q 4 hr × 3 days
	Penicillamine	20 mg/kg/day PO divided q 8 hr
	2,3-dimercaptosuccinic acid (DMSA)	30 mg/kg/day PO tid × 5 days, then 20 mg/kg/day PO bid × 14 days

for occult blood, type and screen/crossmatch, CBC, chemistry, liver function studies, renal studies
- Prevent absorption of iron
  - Lavage
  - Ipecac syrup within first 30 min after ingestion
- Chelation therapy with deferoxamine mesylate
  - A chelation agent is any compound, usually organic, having two or more points of attachment at which an atom of metal may be joined to form a ring-type structure
  - Deferoxamine mesylate forms excretable ferrioxamine complex
  - Deferoxamine dose = 15 mg/kg/hour initial dose
- A change in urine color from pink to orange-red indicates a positive (+) response to chelation therapy
- X-ray will detect undissolved iron tablets in the stomach

ORGANOPHOSPHATE POISONING

- Inhibits acetylcholinesterase
- Absorption is through skin and GI routes
- Produces classic cholinergic syndrome
- SLUDGE mnemonic is indicative of muscarinic symptoms
  - **S** = *S*alivation
  - **L** = *L*acrimation
  - **U** = *U*rination
  - **D** = *D*efecation
  - **G** = *G*I cramping
  - **E** = *E*mesis
- Nicotinic symptoms include motor findings
  - Muscle cramps
  - Weakness
  - Hyperreflexia
  - Fasciculations

- CNS symptoms include
  - Restlessness
  - Ataxia
  - Confusion
  - Coma

ED Treatment

- ABCs
- Decontamination of skin
- Prevent absorption
  - Lavage (do not induce vomiting)
  - Activated charcoal with sorbitol
- Atropine (binds at muscarinic receptors)
  - Dose: 0.05–1.0 mg/kg IV
- Pralidoxime (2-PAM-chloride)
  - Reactivates acetylcholinesterase and reverses cholinergic nicotinic stimulation
  - Given after atropinization
  - Useful if given within 36 hr of exposure
  - Dose: 25–50 mg/kg IV slowly
- Expect tachycardia due to atropinization

PETROLEUM DISTILLATE/ HYDROCARBON EXPOSURE

- Absorbed through GI and skin routes
- Aspiration is a serious problem
- Common ingredient
  - Kerosene
  - Gasoline
  - Napthalene (mothballs)
  - Furniture polish and oils
  - Paint thinner
  - Lighter fluid
  - Turpentine
  - Motor oil
  - Camphor
- High viscosity = limited or low toxicity
- Low viscosity = high toxicity due to possible aspiration

- ***One swallow in a child = approximately 4 mL***
- Cutaneous
  - Eczematoid dermatitis to full-thickness burns
- GI
  - Burns to oropharynx
  - Nausea, vomiting, abdominal pain, diarrhea
- Pulmonary
  - Cyanosis, bronchospasm, wheezing
  - Intercostal and subcostal retractions
  - Hemoptysis, pulmonary edema, fever
- CNS
  - Suppression of ventilatory drive
  - Headache
  - Ataxia
  - Blurred vision
  - Dizziness
  - Lethargy
  - Stupor
  - Coma
- Cardiac
  - Cardiomyopathy
  - Ventricular tachycardia
  - Myocardial injury

ED Treatment

- ABCs
- Supplemental oxygen
- Skin decontamination
- Prevent absorption
  - GI lavage is not indicated unless a large ingestion
- Treat the symptoms
- CHAMP mnemonic for toxic additives
  - **C** = *C*amphor
  - **H** = *H*alogenated hydrocarbons (carbon tetrachloride)
  - **A** = *A*romatic benzenes
  - **M** = *M*etals
  - **P** = *P*esticides

PLANT POISONING

- Many forms of toxic plants are common, often decorative foliage or fruits
  - Children, especially toddlers, put plants, flowers, seeds, pods, berries in mouth
- Common poisonous plants include (but are not limited to)
  - Bird of paradise (pods and seeds)
  - Dumbcane (especially the stem and leaves)
  - Elephant's ears (especially the stem and leaves)
  - English ivy (especially the leaves and berries)
  - Foxglove
  - Holly (berries and leaves)
  - Lily of the valley (all parts)
  - Mistletoe (berries)
  - Poinsettia (all parts)
  - Rhubarb (leaf blades)
  - Peach pits
  - Cherry pits
  - Apricot pits
  - Plum pits
  - Pear seeds
  - Certain mushrooms
- Ingestion is the entry route

Signs and Symptoms

- Oral burning, numbness, or pain
- GI disturbances
- CNS (altered mental status)

ED Treatment

- Dependent on the substance
- ABCs
- GI lavage
- Antihistamines
- Treat the symptoms
- Respiratory support

- Pain control
- Atropine
- Consult your local poison control center for identification and appropriate treatment

SALICYLATE POISONING

- GI absorption through ingestion
- Common ingredient in OTC preparations
- See nomogram for toxicity severity at ingested dose (Fig. 14–2)

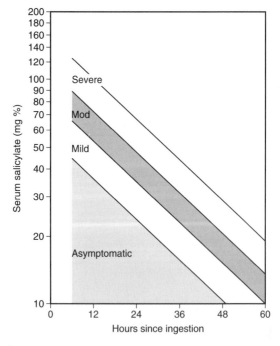

Figure 14–2. Nomogram relating serum salicylate concentration and expected severity of intoxication at varying intervals following the ingestion of a single dose of salicylate. Mod, moderate. (From Done AK: Salicylate intoxication. Pediatrics 26:805, 1960.)

Signs and Symptoms

- Tinnitus
- GI disturbances
- Renal failure
- Tachypnea
- Mental status changes
  - Lethargy
  - Excitability
  - Seizures
  - Coma
- Slurred speech
- Hallucinations
- Systemic collapse
- Allergic reactions

ED Treatment

- ABCs
- Prevent absorption
  - Gastric lavage
  - Activated charcoal with sorbitol (use sorbitol with caution in children)
- Alkalinization of urine pH to 7–8
- Treat any seizures
- Dialysis for renal failure
- A qualitative test for presence of aspirin in urine is to add a few drops of 10% ferric chloride to 5 mL of urine (if aspirin is present, the urine will turn purple in color)

SEDATIVE/HYPNOTIC POISONING

- CNS depressant
- Potentiated by alcohol and/or depressants
- Commonly prescribed drugs
  - Benzodiazepines
    - Alprazolam (Xanax)
    - Lorazepam (Ativan)
    - Diazepam (Valium)

- Alcohol (common additive to cough preparations)
- Meprobamate (Equanil, Miltown)
- Methaqualone (Quaalude)

Signs and Symptoms

- Altered mental status (stupor, coma, seizures)
- Cardiovascular disturbances
  - Arrhythmias
  - Hypotension
- Respiratory depression
- GI disturbances

ED Treatment

- ABCs
- Prevent absorption
  - Lavage
  - Activated charcoal
  - Do not induce vomiting due to rapid onset of CNS side effects
- Flumazenil (Romazicon) is a benzodiazepine receptor antagonist
  - Child dose = 0.01 mg/kg IV (child >20 kg, dosage is 0.2 mg)
  - Adult dose = 0.1–0.3 mg
- Benzodiazepines are the most commonly abused sedative but least likely to cause respiratory depression when used alone (with no other depressants or alcohol)

TRICYCLIC ANTIDEPRESSANT POISONING

- Commonly prescribed for antidepressant therapy and also bedwetting treatment
- Amitriptyline hydrochloride (HCl), doxepin HCl, imipramine HCl, desipramine HCl, nortriptyline HCl, trazodone
- The major toxicity is from anticholinergic and quinidine-like effects
- 10–20 mg/kg can be a toxic ingestion

Signs and Symptoms

- Dry, flushed skin
- Dilated pupils
- Urinary retention
- Dysrythmias due to cardiotoxicity
- Altered LOC
- Seizures
- Coma
- Hypotension (common)

ED Treatment

- ABCs
- EKG
- Pulse oximetry
- Prevent absorption
  - Lavage
  - Activated charcoal with sorbitol
  - Do not induce vomiting due to rapid deterioration and possible loss of airway
- Sodium bicarbonate to maintain blood pH between 7.45 and 7.50
- Respiratory support
- Deterioration is very rapid; expect to intubate as needed

GENERAL TREATMENT

Activated Charcoal Tips

- May be used as a primary gastric decontaminant with or without induced gastric emptying
- May prevent absorption of toxic substance from the gut
  - Must rigorously monitor hydration status
- Ineffective with corrosives and caustic agents, hydrocarbons, alcohol, heavy metals, and water-insoluble compounds

DOSAGES

- Children >12 yr, 50–100 g
- Smaller children, 15–30 g
  - Or 1–2 g/kg is safe and effective
- Activated charcoal is given after lavage or emesis, or alone if ingestion occurred >1 hr before arrival in the ED
- May administer PO or via nasogastric/orogastric tube
- Charcoal can sometimes stain clothing and shoes: Wear personal protective equipment when administering charcoal

Activated Charcoal With Sorbitol

- Children >12 yr, 1 g/kg activated charcoal in 70% sorbitol
- Smaller children, 1 g/kg activated charcoal mixed in 35–70% sorbitol
- Children >1 yr given an initial dose only; subsequent doses of activated charcoal are *without* sorbitol

Whole Bowel Irrigation

- Also known as "gastric decontamination"
- Preferred method to effectively decontaminate the GI tract
- Catharsis alone is ineffective

METHODS

- Syrup of Ipecac
  - Administered within 1–2 hr of ingestion
  - *Never* given if child is lethargic or does not have gag reflex
    - Age 1–5 yr, 15 mL
    - Age 5–12 yr, 30 mL
    - Give 4–8 oz of clear fluid
    - Repeat in 30 min if no vomiting
- Activated charcoal

- See "Activated Charcoal Tips"
- Gastric lavage
  - Use a large-bore orogastric tube
  - Use normal saline to irrigate until the fluid return is clear
  - Child should be in side-lying position with airway protected
- Catharsis
  - Removes coalesced pills (iron ingestion)
  - Use polyethylene glycol (GoLytely)
    - Is a nonabsorbable cathartic
    - Sorbitol and magnesium citrate alone are ineffective

Selected Bibliography

Barkin RM, Rosen P: Emergency Pediatrics, 4th ed. St. Louis, Mosby–Year Book, 1994.

Behrman R, Kliegman R: Nelson Essentials of Pediatrics, 3rd ed. Philadelphia, W.B. Saunders, 1998.

Budassi Sheehy S: Manual of Emergency Care, 3rd ed. St. Louis, C.V. Mosby, 1990.

Chernecky C, Berger B: Laboratory Tests and Diagnostic Procedures, 2nd ed. Philadelphia, W.B. Saunders, 1997.

Emergency Nurses Association: Emergency Nursing Core Curriculum, 4th ed. Philadelphia, W.B. Saunders, 1994.

Fischbach F: A Manual of Laboratory Diagnostic Tests. Philadelphia, J.B. Lippincott, 1980.

Goldfrank L, Flomenbaum N, Lewin N, et al.: Goldfrank's Toxicologic Emergencies, 5th ed. Norwalk, CT, Appleton & Lange, 1994.

Hodgeson B, Kizior R: Saunders Nursing Drug Handbook 1999. Philadelphia, W.B. Saunders, 1999.

Kitt S, Selfridge-Thomas J, Proehl J, Kaiser J: Emergency Nursing: A Physiologic and Clinical Perspective, 2nd ed. Philadelphia, W.B. Saunders, 1995.

Tipsord-Klinkhammer B, Andreoni C: Quick Reference for Emergency Nursing. Philadelphia, W.B. Saunders, 1998.

Chapter 15
Trauma

- Number one killer of children older than 12 mo
- Patterns of injury
  - Head injury is most common form of pediatric trauma
    - Head is proportionately larger than the rest of body until approximately age 10 yr
    - Infants in forward-facing car seats have increased risk of high cervical fractures, as head is projected forward
  - Waddell's triad (Fig. 15–1)
    - Car versus child
      - Initial impact with vehicle: injury to thorax, abdomen, lower extremities
      - Child is thrown from vehicle
      - Child strikes ground head-first
  - Child's height relates to specific injuries when struck by a vehicle
    - Children generally turn toward an oncoming vehicle
    - Toddlers generally knocked down and dragged under vehicle
      - Chest, abdomen, pelvic, femur injuries
    - School-age children generally have femur fractures from impact with bumper

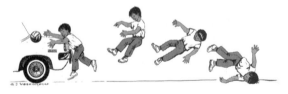

Figure 15–1. Waddell's triad of injuries. (From Wong L: Whaley and Wong's Nursing Care of Infants and Children, 5th ed. St. Louis, Mosby–Year Book, 1995, p. 327.)

- Chest injury from hood of vehicle
- Head injury from striking windshield
- Considerations in motor vehicle crashes
  - Use of restraint/type of restraint used
  - Position/placement of child in vehicle
  - Type of vehicle
  - Speed of each vehicle involved
  - Angle of impact

THE AIRWAY, BREATHING, AND CIRCULATION (ABCs) OF PEDIATRIC TRAUMA CARE

Primary Assessment

- A+ = Airway (plus simultaneous cervical spine immobilization)
  - Assess
    - Patency of airway
      - Tongue is proportionately larger; places child at risk for obstruction
  - Interventions
    - Manual maneuvers to open airway
      - Jaw thrust or chin lift
      - Maintain head in neutral position; avoid excessive flexion or hyperextension
    - Remove loose foreign materials
    - Suction
    - Airway adjuncts
      - Nasal airway
      - Oral airway
        - Use tongue blade to depress tongue and insert without rotation
        - Insertion with rotation of oral airway can cause damage to mucous membranes, soft palate
          - Tissue damage, bleeding can obstruct airway
    - Stabilize cervical spine
      - Neutral position, towel rolls, tape to backboard

- Apply properly fitting rigid collar
- B = Breathing
  - Assess
    - Presence or absence of spontaneous respirations
    - Quality of respirations
      - Respiratory rate (RR), depth, symmetry, accessory muscles, retractions, nasal flaring, head bobbing, grunting
    - Breath sounds
    - Open chest wounds, surface trauma
      - Bruising, abrasions, pattern injury (i.e., tire treads), lacerations, avulsions
    - Muscle tone
    - Level of consciousness (LOC)
  - Interventions
    - Provide 100% FIO_2
      - Bag-valve-mask (BVM) or non-rebreather mask at 12–15 L/min of oxygen
      - Gastric tube insertion necessary to decompress stomach when BVM used
    - Monitor pulse oximetry and heart rate (HR)
      - Hypoxia may be evidenced by decreasing HR
    - Prepare for and assist with intubation
      - Indicated whenever child unable to protect own airway, maintain oxygenation or ventilation
        - In young children, the glottic opening is higher and more anterior
        - Narrowest part of airway is at cricoid ring (not vocal cords)
          - Use uncuffed endotracheal tube for children ≤8 yr
        - Trachea is shorter; depth of insertion is less than that for older children and adults
      - Consider rapid sequence intubation
      - Oral intubation is preferred in children
      - Preoxygenate with 100% FIO_2 for 2–5 min (BVM or non-rebreather mask)

- Maintain cervical spine in neutral position
- Monitor HR and SpO_2
- Apply cricoid pressure (Sellick maneuver) to lessen risk of aspiration
- Confirm placement
  - Check breath sounds laterally and over apices
  - Ascertain absence of breath sounds over stomach
  - Observe symmetric chest rise and fall
  - Use of pediatric end-tidal carbon dioxide detector (pediatric device if >2 kg and <15 kg)
  - Chest x-ray (CXR)
- Prepare for chest tube insertion as indicated by child's condition (see Section VII, Procedure 1 Insertion of Chest Tube)
- C = Circulation
  - Assess
    - Presence and quality of pulses
      - Central and peripheral
      - Rate, strength
    - Skin signs
      - Color, temperature, moisture
    - Capillary refill—interventions necessary if >2 sec
    - LOC
    - Obvious external bleeding
      - Approximate circulating blood volumes
        - Neonate 85–90 mL/kg
        - Infant 75–80 mL/kg
        - Child 70–75 mL/kg
        - Adult 65–70 mL/kg
    - Blood pressure (BP)
      - Hypotension due to hypovolemia is a late sign
      - Hypotension indicates a loss of at least 25% circulating blood volume (see Section I, Reference 25 Classification of Hemorrhagic Shock in Pediatric Trauma

Patients Based on Systemic Signs and Normal Pediatric Vital Signs)
- Interventions
  - CPR as indicated with pediatric advanced life support measures
  - Direct pressure to external bleeding sites
  - Initiate two large-bore (22 gauge or larger) IV lines
    - Initiate intraosseous (IO) infusion if unable to obtain IV access within 90 sec or after three attempts (see Section VII, Procedure 5 Intraosseous Infusion, and Procedure 10 Peripheral IV Insertion)
    - Administer 20 mL/kg IV/IO bolus of warmed 0.9% sodium chloride or lactated Ringer's solution as rapidly as possible (see Section VII, Procedure 7 IV Fluid Bolus Administration)
      - Use stopcock with syringe as close to administration site as possible to "push" fluids in rapidly
      - Reassess child after first bolus
      - May repeat fluid bolus two times if reassessments indicate need
      - For inadequate perfusion after boluses, administer blood
        - 10 mL/kg crossmatched (or type-specific) packed red blood cells
        - 20 mL/kg O negative whole blood
  - Obtain blood for diagnostic testing
    - "Trauma panel"—stat hemoglobin and hematocrit, glucose, type and crossmatch, toxicology screen, electrolytes
- D = Disability
  - Assess
    - LOC—Use "AVPU"
      - **A**lert
      - Responds to **V**erbal stimuli
      - Responds to **P**ainful stimuli
      - **U**nresponsive to any stimuli
    - Activity level

- Pupillary assessment
- Interventions
  - Glucose—documented hypoglycemia
  - Naloxone—suspected narcotic overdose
  - Flumazenil—suspected benzodiazepine overdose

Secondary Assessment

- E = Expose
  - Expose child completely, cut off all clothing
- F = Farenheit
  - Children have proportionately larger body surface area
    - More susceptible to heat loss
    - Hypothermia/cold stress may make resuscitation efforts less successful
  - Monitor temperature
  - Maintain normothermia
    - Warm blankets
    - Radiant warmer
    - Overhead heat lamps
    - Warmed IV fluids and blood products
    - Increased temperature of resuscitation room
- G = Get
  - Get a full set of vital signs (BP, HR, RR, rectal temperature)
  - Get the child on monitors
    - Cardiac monitor with RR and apnea alarm function
    - Noninvasive BP monitor or arterial line monitoring
    - Pulse oximetry
    - End-tidal capnography, if available
    - Temperature, continuous core temperature monitoring if hypothermic
  - Get tubes in place
    - Gastric tube
      - Indicated for child who has been intubated, has abdominal trauma, is unresponsive, or with multisystem trauma

- Indwelling urinary catheter
  - All children who have multisytem trauma who have required fluid resuscitation
  - Urinary output is an important evaluation of the effectiveness of resuscitation efforts
  - Assess for blood at urinary meatus or other signs of perineal area bleeding prior to insertion
  - Dipstick urine specimen for presence of blood; send for urinalysis, possibly toxicology screen and pregnancy testing
- H^1 = History
  - Mechanism of injury
    - Vehicular crash
      - Position in vehicle, type and use of restraint, speed, angle of impact
    - Fall—height fallen from
      - Significant fall = three times the child's height
      - Children most often land on head, back
  - Treatment prior to arrival in the emergency department
  - AMPLE history components
    - **A**llergies
    - **M**edications
    - **P**ast medical history
      - Birth history
    - **L**ast oral intake/meal
    - **E**vents leading up to the injury
  - Immunization status
- H^2 = Head-to-toe assessment
  - Collect data by use of inspection, auscultation, palpation, percussion
  - Consider congruence of history and physical findings as they relate to possible child maltreatment
  - Perform systemic assessment from head to lower extremities, including posterior surfaces
  - Head/face/neck

- Anterior and posterior fontanels in infants
- Periorbital ecchymosis (raccoon's eyes)
- Ecchymosis over mastoid process (Battle's sign)
- Asymmetry, step defects, palpable deformities
- Subcutaneous emphysema
- Surface trauma
- Chest
  - Respiratory effort
  - Breath sounds and heart sounds
  - Chest wall tenderness
  - Surface trauma
- Abdomen
  - Bowel sounds in all quadrants
  - Abdominal tenderness, distention, rigidity
  - Surface trauma
- Pelvis/genitalia
  - Pelvic stability
  - Blood at urinary meatus
  - Perineal area bleeding
  - Surface trauma
- Extremities
  - Deformity
  - Distal circulation, motor function, sensation (CMS)
  - Surface trauma
- Posterior assessment
  - Maintain spinal immobilization
    - Log roll the child
  - Deformities, tenderness to palpation
  - Surface trauma
- I = Interventions
  - In addition to those previously mentioned
  - Pain control measures
    - Distraction, family presence
    - Comfort measures, positioning, warmth
    - Administration of analgesics
  - Initiate and maintain NPO status
  - Involve family in child's care as appropriate
  - Stabilize—do not remove—impaled objects
  - Tetanus immunization as indicated

Additional Diagnostic Considerations

- Trauma radiographs for multisystem trauma
  - Cross-table lateral cervical spine
  - Complete cervical spine series
  - Chest
  - Abdomen
  - Pelvis
  - Extremities and others as indicated
- Computed tomographic (CT) scan
  - Brain—head injury
  - Abdomen—abdominal assessment of child often unreliable
    - CT scan of abdomen with contrast will detect majority of injuries to liver, spleen, and kidneys
- Diagnostic peritoneal lavage (DPL)
  - Rarely used in children
    - Most blunt abdominal injuries are treated medically
    - Possible indications for DPL
      - Child going to surgery for another procedure without CT of abdomen; abdominal injury suspected
      - Critically injured child to be rapidly transferred to tertiary care facility; DPL may indicate need for surgical procedure prior to transfer
- Calculate Pediatric (Modified) Glasgow Coma Scale score (see Section I, Reference 13 Pediatric Modification of Glasgow Coma Scale by Age of Patient)
- Calculate Pediatric Trauma Score (see Section I, Reference 22 Pediatric Trauma Score)

PENETRATING TRAUMA

- Underlying tissues are damaged in the path of the wounding instrument or missile
- Stab wounds

- Consider
  - Length of instrument
  - Angle of entry into the tissue
  - Velocity of stabbing force
  - Multiple body cavities of a child may be penetrated by a single stab wound
  - Damage to adjacent structures out of direct path of stab wound may be present, resulting from disruption and displacement of tissue during injury
- Firearm injuries
  - Consider
    - Projectile mass, shape, size, and composition
    - Type of tissue penetrated
    - Velocity of bullet (depends on distance)
      - Low-velocity missiles (<1000 ft/sec) (handguns) cause little cavitation or blast effect
      - Low-energy transfer to tissues
      - High-velocity missiles (>3000 ft/sec) (rifles) compress and accelerate tissue away from the bullet
      - Create a cavity with negative pressure behind the missile
      - Debris contaminates the wound
      - High-energy transfer
    - Density
      - The greater the tissue density, the more energy/damage to the tissue

CHEST TRAUMA

- Most common presentation is hypoxemia and increased respiratory effort
- Pneumothorax
  - Most common form of pediatric chest trauma
  - Accumulation of air in pleural space
  - Diminished, absent, or altered breath sounds over injured side
    - Infants and young children transmit breath

      sounds over thorax due to less subcutaneous tissue/thin thoracic wall; absence of breath sounds may not be evident on auscultation
- Obtain CXR
- Prepare for and assist with chest tube insertion (see Section VII, Procedure 1 Insertion of Chest Tube)

- Tension pneumothorax
  - Trapped air in pleural space cannot escape; places pressure on lung, mediastinal structures, great vessels
  - Venous return to the heart is compromised
  - Cardiac output is decreased
  - Signs and symptoms
    - Decreased air entry and bulging of chest over injured side
    - Severe respiratory distress
    - Older children: tracheal deviation to the opposite side and jugular vein distention
  - Prepare for and assist with immediate needle thoracostomy and insertion of chest tube
    - Needle insertion at second intercostal space midclavicular line, affected side (see Section VII, Procedure 1 Insertion of Chest Tube)

- Hemothorax
  - Because of smaller circulating blood volumes in children, a "small" blood loss into the thorax may result in signs and symptoms of shock
  - Signs and symptoms include signs of decreased perfusion and respiratory distress
  - Prepare for and assist with chest tube insertion and fluid volume resuscitation (see Section VII, Procedure 1 Insertion of Chest Tube)

ABDOMINAL TRAUMA

- Children at increased risk for abdominal trauma

- Abdominal muscles not well developed
- Chest wall less protective than sturdy adult thoracic cage
- Liver and spleen less protected
- Increased vascular supply of duodenum
- Abdominal examination in young children is often unreliable
- Liver and spleen injuries
  - Splenic injuries most common
    - Sports injury, fall from bicycle, motor vehicle crash
    - Nonoperative, conservative management is first choice
  - Liver lacerations are a major cause of morbidity and mortality
  - Serial assessments necessary for both liver and spleen injury
    - Abdominal girth, hemoglobin and hematocrit, vital signs and perfusion

Selected Bibliography

Emergency Nurses Association: Emergency Nursing Pediatric Course Instructor Manual. Park Ridge, IL, Emergency Nurses Association, 1993.

Singh N: Manual of Pediatric Critical Care. Philadelphia, W.B. Saunders, 1997.

Soud TE, Rogers JS: Manual of Pediatric Emergency Nursing. St. Louis, Mosby–Year Book, 1998.

Tipsord-Klinkhammer B, Andreoni C: Quick Reference for Emergency Nursing. Philadelphia, W.B. Saunders, 1998.

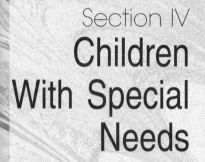

Section IV
Children
With Special
Needs

CHILDREN AND MECHANICAL VENTILATION

- Respiratory failure can be a result of
  - Head injury
  - Spinal cord injury
  - Congenital defects
  - Neuromuscular disease states
  - Bronchopulmonary dysplasia (BPD)
- Tracheostomy is common in children with long-term ventilation
- Types of mechanical ventilators
  - Pressure-cycled
  - Volume-cycled
  - High-frequency ventilators
    - High-frequency positive-pressure ventilation
    - High-frequency jet ventilation
    - High-frequency oscillation
- Modes of ventilation
  - Continuous mandatory ventilation (CMV)
  - Assist-control ventilation (ACV)
  - Intermittent mandatory ventilation (IMV)
  - Synchronized intermittent mandatory ventilation (SIMV)
  - Pressure-support ventilation (PSV)
  - Pressure-controlled inverse ratio ventilation (PC-IRV)
  - Airway pressure release ventilation (APRV)
  - Synchronous independent lung ventilation (SILV)
- Adjuncts to mechanical ventilation
  - Positive end-expiratory pressure (PEEP)
    - Maintains positive pressure at end of expiration
    - Increases functional residual capacity (FRC)
    - Keeps open and/or inflates collapsed alveoli
  - Continuous positive airway pressure (CPAP)
    - For larger, older children breathing spontaneously

- • Can adequately ventilate, but cannot effectively oxygenate because of decreased FRC
  - • Can help patients with secretions blocking the airway or with fluid-filled alveoli
  - • Can also be used to treat refractory hypoxemia resulting from atelectasis
  - • A tight-fitting, continuous-flow face mask is necessary
  - • Careful assessment of cardiovascular and ventilatory status during CPAP is required
  - • Consider insertion of nasogastric (NG) tube to decrease risk of gastric dilatation, vomiting, and aspiration
  - • Usually tolerated for 12–36 hr
- • Troubleshooting ventilators (Table IV–1)
- • Suctioning
  - • Airway must remain patent
  - • Mucous plugs can occlude lumen of tracheostomy tube or endotracheal tube
    - • Hyperventilate with 100% oxygen before and after suctioning

Table IV–1. Troubleshooting Ventilators

Problem	Intervention
Pressure alarm	Assess for plugged/occluded tube
	Suction airway for secretions
	Empty condensation fluid
	Assess for kinked tubing
	Reposition the patient
	Insert oral airway
	Assess for hypoxia or bronchospasm
	Adjust sensitivity
	Assess patient's need for sedation
Volume alarm	Assess for leak in endotracheal tube cuff
	Assess for leak or disconnection in ventilator tubing

- Use a suction catheter that is half the size of the tracheostomy or endotracheal tube
- Use aseptic technique
- Suction for no more than 3–4 sec
- Prevent hypoxia
- Allow child to rest for 30–60 sec between suctioning
- Signs of tube occlusion
  - Tachycardia
  - Increased respiratory rate
  - A fall in oxygen saturation

CHILDREN WITH DEVELOPMENTAL DELAYS

- Mental retardation (MR)
  - Classified by IQ
    - Mild—IQ 50–55 to ~70
    - Moderate—IQ 35–40 to ~50–55
    - Severe—IQ 20–25 to ~35–40
    - Profound—IQ <20–25
  - Screening tests
    - Denver Developmental Screening Test (DDST)
      - Screens development of children from birth to age 6 yr
    - The Denver II
    - Early Language Milestone (ELM)
    - The Carey Infant Temperament Questionnaire
      - Assesses temperament in infants 4–8 mo old
    - Brazelton Neonatal Behavioral Assessment Scale
    - Pediatrics Examination of Educational Readiness
    - Pediatric Early Elementary Examination
    - Stanford-Binet, Wechsler, Bayley Scales of Infant Development
    - Vineland Adaptive Behavior Scales
  - Children with developmental delays may have other syndromes or dysfunctions

- Children present to the emergency department with the same acute illness, injury, or complications of chronic illness
- Inclusion of parent/caregiver is important
- Speak to child as though he or she can understand
- Protect the child's safety needs

Selected Bibliography

Aswill J, Droske S: Nursing Care of Children: Principles and Practice. Philadelphia, W.B. Saunders, 1997.

Behrman R, Kliegman R: Nelson Essentials of Pediatrics, 3rd ed. Philadelphia, W.B. Saunders, 1998.

Betz C, Sowden L: Mosby's Pediatric Nursing Reference, 3rd ed. St. Louis, Mosby–Year Book, 1996.

Kelly W (ed): Respiratory Support. Springhouse, PA, Springhouse Corporation, 1991.

Soud T, Rogers J: Manual of Pediatric Emergency Nursing. St. Louis, Mosby–Year Book, 1998.

Tipsord-Klinkhammer B, Andreoni C: Quick Reference for Emergency Nursing. Philadelphia, W.B. Saunders, 1998.

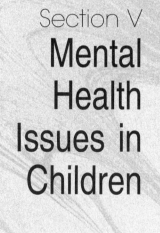

Mental Health Issues in Children

DEPRESSION

- Dysthymic disorder
  - Depressed or irritable mood >1 yr
- Bipolar mood disorder
  - Highs and lows—mood swings for ≥1 yr
- Major depressive disorder
  - ≥2 wk of depressed, irritable mood
  - Sleep disturbances
  - Loss of appetite
  - Lethargy
  - Disturbance of self-esteem
- Genetics and ineffective parenting thought to be the basis for affective disorders
- Depression before adolescence is rare but does occur
  - Incidence is 0.4–6.4%

Signs and Symptoms

- Fatigue
- Insomnia or hypersomnia
- Feelings of sadness
- Irritability
- Somatic complaints without physical findings
- Sadness or gloominess
- Weight loss or weight gain
- Poor self-esteem
- Substance abuse
- Suicidal ideation
  - Suicide is the leading cause of death in adolescents
  - Warning signs
    - Stated suicide plan
    - Significant loss
    - Significant family event
    - Close friends with "suicide pact"
    - Frequent "accidents"
    - A history of bulimia nervosa
      - 5% of persons with bulimia nervosa commit suicide

- Sad Persons Suicide Risk Assessment
  - **S** = **S**ex
  - **A** = **A**ge
  - **D** = **D**epression
  - **P** = **P**revious attempts
  - **E** = **E**thanol
  - **R** = **R**ational thinking loss
  - **S** = **S**ocial supports lacking
  - **O** = **O**rganized plan
  - **N** = **N**o spouse (or significant other)
  - **S** = **S**ickness

Emergency Department (ED) Treatment

- Airway, breathing, and circulation (ABCs)
- Assess for suicide risk
- Psychiatric evaluation as indicated
- Provide a safe environment
  - Remove sharps, shoestrings, belts, wastebasket plastic liner bags
- Medical clearance examination
  - Usually includes alcohol and drug screening
  - Electrocardiogram if cocaine use suspected or acknowledged
- Hospital admission includes suicide precautions
- Possible discharge home with outpatient treatment if suicide risk is low or absent and a responsible parent/caregiver is able and willing to monitor child closely

SUBSTANCE ABUSE

- Two thirds of teens experiment with illicit drugs before age 18 yr
- 5% of high school seniors
  - Smoke cigarettes daily
  - Drink alcohol daily
  - Smoke cigarettes *and* drink alcohol daily
    - Experimental use of alcohol and tobacco

can lead to further drug experimentation and/or addiction
- Cigarettes and alcohol are considered "gateway" drugs
- Smokeless tobacco
  - Nicotine is addictive
- "Dipping" can lead to oral cancers

Classification of Substance Abuse

- Nonuse
- Experimental
- Recreational
- Circumstantial
- Habitual
- Compulsive

Alcohol

- Signs and symptoms
  - Flushing of skin
  - Tachycardia
  - Increased sweating
  - Mydriasis
  - Dysarthria
  - Incoordination
  - Change in level of consciousness
  - Emotional lability
  - Impaired cardiac output
  - Arrhythmias
  - Nausea and vomiting
  - Coma
  - Death
- ED treatment
  - ABCs
    - Anticipate support of ventilation as indicated
  - Alcohol level (blood or breath)
  - Drug screen as indicated
  - Systemic monitoring, including pulse oximetry as indicated

- IV access
- Fluid replacement
- Glucose and thiamine as indicated

Cocaine

- Multisystem effects
  - Tachycardia
  - Bradycardia
  - Arrhythmias
  - Angina
  - Myocardial infarction
  - Endocarditis
  - Hypertension
  - Bronchitis, pneumonia
  - Pneumothorax
  - Pulmonary edema
  - Vasculitis
  - Deep vein thrombosis
  - Weight loss
  - Hyperthermia
  - Epistaxis
  - Ulcerations
  - Septal perforation
  - Sinusitis
  - Nausea and vomiting
  - Abdominal pain
  - Coke burns
  - Phlebitis
- ED treatment
  - ABCs
  - IV access
  - Drug screen
  - Systemic monitoring, including pulse oximetry
  - Cooling measures for hyperthermia
  - Anticipate possible seizures
    - Diazepam IV
    - Padded stretcher
  - Nitroprusside, labetalol for hypertension

Lysergic Acid Diethylamide (LSD)

- Signs and symptoms
  - Hallucinations
    - Visual
    - Auditory
    - Tactile
    - Olfactory
  - Agitation
  - Dysphoria
  - Hypertension
  - Tachycardia
  - Hyperthermia
- ED treatment
  - ABCs
  - IV access
  - Drug screen
  - Systemic monitoring, including pulse oximetry as indicated
  - Reassurance
  - May require haloperidol injection

Marijuana

- Signs and symptoms
  - Euphoria
  - Elation
  - Relaxation
  - Dreaminess
  - Laughing or silliness
  - Impaired judgment and thought processes
  - Altered concepts of time, space, body image
  - Speech changes
  - Chest tightness
  - Head pressure
  - Increased appetite and/or thirst
  - Ataxia
  - Tremors
  - Tachycardia
- ED treatment
  - ABCs

- Drug screen
- Treat the symptoms
- Supportive, nonjudgmental environment

Opioids

- Signs and symptoms
  - Respiratory depression
  - Central nervous system depression
  - Hypotension
  - Bradycardia
  - Skin abscess
  - Osteomyelitis
  - Nephritis
  - Hepatitis
  - HIV
- ED treatment
  - ABCs
    - Anticipate support of ventilation as indicated
  - Drug screen
  - IV access
  - Naloxone, 2 mg IV push, repeated up to 10 mg

PCP

- Signs and symptoms
  - Ataxia
  - Nystagmus
  - Hypertension
  - Slurred speech
  - Hallucinations
  - Paranoia
  - Confusion
  - Convulsions
  - Flashbacks
  - Death related to successful suicide or accidents
  - Extreme physical strength
- ED treatment

- ABCs
- IV access as indicated
- Drug screen
- May require haloperidol and/or diazepam for psychosis or convulsions
- Padded hard restraints if indicated
  - Follow your institution's policy and procedure
- Maintain patient safety

EATING DISORDERS

Anorexia Nervosa

- Affects 1–5% of teenage girls
- 20:1 female-to-male ratio
- Hallmarks
  - Pleasure in attainment of low weight
    - Weight gain results in severe anxiety
    - Weight loss lessens the anxiety

SIGNS AND SYMPTOMS

- Scalp hair loss
- Lanugo on face and trunk
- Rough, scaly skin
- Petechial rash
- Bradycardia
- Hypotension
- Delayed gastric emptying
- Hypothermia
- Myopathy
- Neuropathy
- Leukopenia
- Malnutrition
- Death if not treated

Bulimia Nervosa

- Affects as many as 5% of female college students
- 10:1 female-to-male ratio

- Hallmarks
  - Binge eating
    - Consumes large quantities of "forbidden food"
    - Consumed rapidly and in secret
    - Taste of the food is not an issue
  - Purge sessions become linked to the binge
    - Self-induced vomiting
      - Possible syrup of ipecac abuse
    - Laxative abuse
    - Diuretic abuse

SIGNS AND SYMPTOMS

- Salivary gland enlargement
- Esophagitis
- Fluid and electrolyte imbalances
- Dental enamel erosion
- Cardiomyopathy
- Malnutrition
- Dizziness
- Syncope
- Constipation
- Menstrual irregularities or absence
- Death if not treated

ED TREATMENT FOR EATING DISORDERS

- ABCs
- Complete blood count, urinalysis, chemistry, urinary chorionic gonadotropin
- IV access
- Electrolyte replacement as indicated
- Psychiatric evaluation
- Hospitalization as required for treatment of severe symptoms

Informational Resources

- National Association of Anorexia Nervosa and Associated Disorders Inc. (ANAD) 847-831-3438

anad20@aol.com; http://members.aol.com/anad20/index.html
* Something Fishy (web site on eating disorders) http://www.somethingfishy.org
* Harvard Eating Disorder Center (HEDC) 888-236-1188
* The American Anorexia/Bulimia Association, Inc. (AA/BA) 212-575-6200

Selected Bibliography

Ashwill J, Droske S: Nursing Care of Children: Principles and Practice. Philadelphia, W.B. Saunders, 1997.

Behrman R, Kliegman R: Nelson Essentials of Pediatrics, 3rd ed. Philadelphia, W.B. Saunders, 1998.

Betz C, Sowden L: Mosby's Pediatric Nursing Reference, 3rd ed. St. Louis, Mosby–Year Book, 1996.

Soud T, Rogers J: Manual of Pediatric Emergency Nursing. St. Louis, Mosby–Year Book, 1998.

Tipsord-Klinkhammer B, Andreoni C: Quick Reference for Emergency Nursing. Philadelphia, W.B. Saunders, 1998.

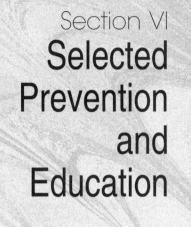

Section VI
Selected Prevention and Education

SAFETY BELT TIPS

- Wear your lap belt low and snug across the hip, and the shoulder belt across your chest
- *Do not* put the shoulder belt under your arm
- Friends don't let friends drive in a car without a seat belt

CAR SAFETY TIPS

- All children are safest in the back seat, using a safety belt or in a child safety seat
- Use a seat belt on every trip, no matter where you are going

BICYCLE SAFETY TIPS

- Ride single file and to the right of the roadway with traffic
- Use hand signals to indicate turns
- Yield to pedestrians
- Never wear headphones while bicycling
- Make sure that your bike has reflectors
- Never give rides on a bicycle meant for one person
- Bicycle helmets—using your head!
  - Children should start using a helmet with their first tricycle
  - Adults should wear a helmet, too—set a good example
  - All professional riders wear helmets!

Intended to be used for patient and family/community education.
This section developed by the 1998 Pediatric Committee of the Illinois State Council, Emergency Nurses Association. Members include Colleen Andreoni, Cathy Collins, Darcy Egging, Harriet Hawkins, Theresa McGuire, Beth Nachtsheim, and Laurie Round. Used with permission.

WHEN ATTENDING A PROFESSIONAL FIREWORKS DISPLAY, KEEP THE FOLLOWING RULES IN MIND

- Obey all ushers or monitors and respect the safety barriers set up
- Resist any temptation to get close to the actual firing site—the best view is from at least a quarter of a mile away
- Leave pets at home—their sensitive ears can be injured by the loud noises
- Fireworks safety
  - Know your state laws regarding the use of specific fireworks
  - Fireworks are not toys—they can cause burn injuries and ignite clothing if used improperly
  - *Never* give fireworks to young children
  - Never experiment or attempt to make your own fireworks

BE SUN SMART AND SUN SAFE

- SPF (sun protection factor) refers to the length of time in the sun to develop a mild sunburn; the higher the number, the greater the protection
- PABA products must be applied 30 min prior to exposure
- Reapply products after swimming or exercise
- Avoid midday sun—it is the strongest
- Clothing is considered a sunscreen—not a sun blocker
- Children, especially infants, burn easily—for best protection, keep them out of the sun
- Keep hats on infants and toddlers

PEDESTRIAN SAFETY TIPS

- Before crossing a street, stop at the curb and look left, right, then left again

- Never let small children cross the street alone
- Always wear bright colors or reflective clothing when walking at night
- Always stay on the sidewalks and crosswalks
- If there are no sidewalks, walk facing traffic
- Cross streets only at intersections
- Make eye contact with the driver when crossing busy streets

SWIMMING SAFELY

- Do not go into deep water with a raft or flotation toy
- Children under 3 yr old should never be left alone in a wading pool or a bathtub
- Never leave children unattended near a swimming pool
- First, learn to swim!
- Never permit anyone to swim alone
- Do not dive into shallow water
- Swim only in supervised areas
- Swim with a buddy

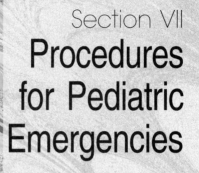

Section VII
Procedures for Pediatric Emergencies

Procedure 1
Insertion of Chest Tube

INDICATIONS

- Removal of air or liquid from the pleural space
  - May be a result of trauma, disease, or spontaneous event
  - Hemothorax
    - Massive hemothorax is rare in children
  - Pneumothorax
  - Tension pneumothorax
  - Empyema (generally nonemergent)
  - Prophylactic placement in chest trauma patients who require positive-pressure ventilation (usually due to flail chest)

SUPPLIES

- Cardiac monitor
- Pulse oximeter
- Supplemental oxygen
- Consider nasogastric or orogastric tube to aid in stomach decompression
- Analgesia as ordered
- Sterile field
  - Gloves and mask
- Local anesthesia
- Chest tube insertion tray or commercial kit
- Consider use of autotransfusion collection chamber if massive hemothorax suspected
- Chest tube size dependent on age (Table P1–1)
- Suction
- Dressing material and tape
  - May use biooclusive dressing

Table P1–1. Chest Tube Sizes and Suction Pressure for Pediatrics		
Age	Tube Size (French)	cm H$_2$O
Infant	10–14	10
Child 1–3 yr	16–20	20
Child 4–7 yr	20–24	20
Child 8–12 yr	28–32	20
Child ≥13 yr	≥28	20

PROCEDURE

- Wash hands
- Apply gloves
- Maintain universal precautions
- Sedation or analgesia as indicated
- After chest tube is placed, monitor
  - Cardiac status
  - Pulse oximetry
  - Fluctuation in tube
  - Output
  - Color of fluid (if any)
  - Air leaks
    - Air leaks can occur as follows
      - From chest drainage system
      - Continued air leak in the lung
      - Esophageal or bronchial injury
      - Incorrectly positioned chest tube
- Tape all tube connections
- Obtain specimens of chest tube drainage only from the collection port on the system
- Clamping of chest tube during transport not necessary; a tension pneumothorax may develop if the chest tube is clamped before re-expansion of the lung
- Observe for
  - Subcutaneous emphysema
  - Occlusion of chest drainage tubing from kinks or clots

Procedure 2
Conscious Sedation

INDICATIONS

- Procedures that are painful but relatively short in duration; i.e., fracture reduction, extensive suturing/wound repair, débridement
- Pharmacologic agents include analgesics and sedatives
- The child under "conscious sedation"
  - Has a decreased level of consciousness (LOC)
  - Maintains protective reflexes
  - Maintains a patent airway independently
  - Responds appropriately to physical or verbal stimuli
- Routes of administration may include IV, IM, sublingual, inhalation, and oral
- The child requires continuous monitoring during sedation until return to presedation level: heart rate, blood pressure (BP), respiratory rate, pulse oximetry, and LOC
- Emergency equipment: drugs, airway and ventilatory equipment, defibrillator, and O_2 must be immediately accessible

SUPPLIES

- Medication as ordered
- Specific reversal agents for sedation medications
- Bag-valve-mask device appropriate for child's size
- Oxygen non-rebreather mask, oxygen nasal cannula

- Working suction with suction catheters and tonsil suction
- Intubation equipment of appropriate size
- Cardiorespiratory monitor
- Pulse oximeter
- Noninvasive BP (NIBP) cuff and monitor
- Documentation tools at bedside

PROCEDURE

- Explain the procedure to the child and parents—consider age and developmental level
- Review and/or witness informed consent for procedure (physician explains procedure to the parents and obtains the informed consent)
- Wash hands
- Establish a peripheral IV line
- Connect child to cardiorespiratory monitor, pulse oximeter, and NIBP monitor
  - Obtain and document presedation vital signs
  - Set monitors to obtain data every 5–15 min during sedation and procedure
    - Review institutional policy regarding specific documentation requirements during procedure
- Administer the sedation and analgesics as ordered; in many institutions this is a physician role—review your own policy and procedure
  - See Table P2–1 for medications frequently used
- Continuously observe the child during the sedation
  - Chest is uncovered to promote visualization of respirations
  - Child is positioned to maintain airway patency
  - Monitors and the child's LOC are continuously observed
  - Oxygen by nasal cannula may be administered during the procedure at the physician's discretion

Table P2-1. Drugs Commonly Used for Conscious Sedation

Drug	Dosage	Actions	Nursing Considerations
Benzodiazepines Midazolam (Versed)	Dosage must be individualized and titrated Administer IV dose over 2–5 min Additional doses are in increments of 25% of initial dose after waiting an additional 2 min to evaluate effect IV: 0.035–0.15 mg/kg Maximum dose: 4 mg PO: 0.25–1.0 mg/kg Maximum dose: 20 mg Nasal: 0.2–0.5 mg/kg Maximum dose: 5 mg Rectal: 0.3–0.5 mg/kg	IV: Onset, 1–5 min Duration, 15–20 min PO: Onset, 10–20 min Duration, up to 3 hr Nasal: Onset, 5 min Peak, 10 min Duration, 30–60 min Rectal: Onset, 20–30 min Peak, 20 min	Depresses subcortical levels of CNS Rapid IV administration may lead to apnea Minimal analgesia Excellent hypnotic/sedative Excellent amnesia Used alone or with an opiate Dilute with 0.9 sodium chloride to a 1 mg/mL formulation to facilitate slower IV injection Three to four times as potent as diazepam Transient apnea has been seen with doses of 0.15 mg/kg Oral concentration: 2 mg/mL Do not repeat oral dose

Drug	Dosage	Onset/Duration	Comments
Diazepam (Valium)	Dosage should be titrated to desired sedative effect IV: 0.2–0.3 mg/kg Do not exceed 1–2 mg/min IVP Maximum dose: 10 mg PO: 0.2–0.5 mg/kg Maximum dose: 20 mg Rectal: 0.5 mg/kg Maximum dose: 10 mg	IV: Onset, 1–5 min PO: Onset, 30 min Duration, 2–3 hr Rectal: Onset, 10 min Duration, 1–2 hr	Depresses subcortical levels of CNS Incompatible with all solutions in syringe—do not dilute Observe for respiratory depression
Lorazepam (Ativan)	IV: 0.02–0.05 mg/kg Slow IV (2 mg/min) Maximum dose: 2 mg	IV: Onset, 10 min Duration, up to 8 hr	Depresses subcortical levels of CNS Dilute medication with equal amount of compatible solution to facilitate slow IV injection
Barbiturates Thiopental (Pentothal)	IV: 2 mg/kg Rectal suspension < 3 mo: 15 mg/kg MR a 7.5 mg dose after 15 min Child: 25 mg/kg MR a 15 mg/kg dose after 15 min Do *not* give more than one initial and one repeated dose in 24 hr	IV: Onset, 30–40 sec Duration, 5–30 min Rectal: Onset, 3–5 min Duration, >30 min	Acts in reticular-activating system to produce anesthesia Relatively long-acting NPO 3 hr prior to rectal dose For rectal dose, adjust down to nearest 50 mg increment for accurate measurement No analgesic effects Respiratory depression, bronchospasm Caution in asthma and increased ICP

Table continued on following page

321

Table P2–1. Drugs Commonly Used for Conscious Sedation *Continued*

Drug	Dosage	Actions	Nursing Considerations
Opiates Morphine	IV: 0.1–0.2 mg/kg Maximum: 10 mg/dose IM: 0.1–0.2 mg/kg Maximum: 15 mg/dose SQ: 0.1–0.2 mg/kg	IV: Onset, 5–6 min Peak, 20 min Duration, 4–5 hr IM: Peak, 30–60 min Duration, 4–5 hr SQ: Onset, 15–30 min Peak, 50–90 min Duration, 4–5 hr	Depresses pain impulse transmission Respiratory depression Dilute medication with compatible solution to a 1 mg/mL formulation to facilitate slower IV injection Caution in asthma, increased ICP
Fentanyl (Sublimaze)	IV/IM: 1–3 µg/kg Give slowly over 3–5 min Transmucosal/oral lollipop: 10–15 µg/kg	IV: Onset, immediate to 5 min Peak, 3–5 min Duration, 30–60 min IM: Onset, 7–15 min Peak, 30 min Duration, 1–2 hr Transmucosal: Onset, 5–15 min Peak, 20–35 min Duration, 1–2 hr	Inhibits ascending pain pathway in CNS, increases pain threshold, alters pain perception 100 times more potent than morphine Both sedative and analgesic properties Bradycardia, respiratory depression, "frozen chest" (chest muscle rigidity), and hypotension associated with too-rapid IVP or excessive dose
Others Ketamine	IV: 1–2 mg/kg Maximum dose: 100 mg Give IVP over 1 min	IV: Onset, immediate Peak, 1 min Duration, 15 min	Phencyclidine derivative Acts on limbic system cortex to produce anesthesia

Drug	Dose	Onset/Duration	Comments
	Supplemental doses at 0.5 mg/kg IM: 1–5 mg/kg Maximum dose: 50 mg Rectal: 5–10 mg/kg Nasal: 3–5 mg/kg Sublingual: 3–5 mg/kg	IM: Onset, 30–60 min Duration, 1 hr	Sedation, analgesia, and amnesic effects Trance-like state, catalepsy, nystagmus Increased secretions May give atropine 0.01 mg/kg 10 min prior to dose Contraindicated in head injury/increased ICP Dilute in equal amount of compatible solution to facilitate slow IV injection
Chloral hydrate	Rectal: 50–75 mg/kg Oral: 50–75 mg/kg Maximum dose: 1 g MR dose once	Rectal/oral: Onset, 20–30 min Duration, 4–12 hr	No analgesic effects Prolonged sedation and hypoventilation at high doses
Reversal Agents			
Flumazenil (Romazicon)	IV: 5–10 µg/kg/dose Give over 15 sec MR every 1 min, up to maximum of 1–3 mg/hr	IV: Onset, 1–2 min Peak, 6–10 min Duration, >30 min Resedation may occur within 1 hr	Benzodiazepine receptor antagonist Reverses sedation effects of benzodiazepines
Naloxone (Narcan)	IV: 0.01–0.1 mg/kg/dose May also give IM, SQ, ET	IV: Onset, immediate to 2 min Duration, 30–40 min Resedation may occur within 1 hr	Narcotic antagonist

CNS, central nervous system; ET, via endotracheal tube; ICP, intracranial pressure; IVP, IV push; MR, may repeat.

- Remain with the child after the procedure until the effects of the medication have worn off
- Document postprocedure return to baseline vital signs and LOC
  - Prior to discharge, the child should be
    - Awake and alert
    - Able to sit up unsupported
    - Able to drink fluids
    - Able to speak clearly (if age appropriate)

Procedure 3
Defibrillation and Cardioversion

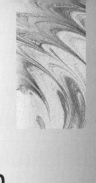

INDICATIONS (Table P3–1)

- Defibrillation is used for restoration of organized electrical activity, which should result in organized myocardial contraction
  - Utilizes asynchronous electrical current
- Cardioversion is used for tachydysrhythmias that have become symptomatic
  - Utilizes synchronized electrical current that coincides with the patient's myocardial electrical activity

SUPPLIES

- A standard defibrillator with synchronous mode for cardioversion

Table P3–1. Pediatric Defibrillation and Cardioversion

Weight (kg)	Defibrillation (J)	Cardioversion (J)
4	8–16	2–4
6	12–24	3–6
8	16–32	4–8
10	20–40	5–10
15	30–60	8–15
20	40–80	10–20
30	60–120	15–30
40	80–160	20–40
50	100–200	25–50

- Defibrillation pads, patches, cream, paste, or saline pads
  - Do not use alcohol pads or ultrasound gel
- Monitoring capability (may be through the paddles, defibrillation/monitoring-type patches, or via separate cable)
- Infant paddles for children up to 10 kg
  - Many defibrillators have infant paddles under "slide off" adult paddles, or they may have a separate cable connection
- Adult paddles for children >10 kg
- If defibrillation is required, other resuscitative measures will be in use (airway, IV access, medications)
- If cardioversion is required, consider sedation as indicated

PROCEDURE

- Observe universal precautions
- Consider sedation for cardioversion
- Apply defibrillation pads, patches, cream, paste, or saline pads
- Apply paddles to chest
  - One paddle is placed at the right upper chest below the clavicle
  - One paddle is placed at the left chest in the anterior axillary line left of the nipple
  - May use anterior-posterior paddle placement as indicated
  - Apply paddles with enough pressure to overcome transthoracic resistance
  - Choose correct joule setting for either defibrillation or cardioversion
- Observe safety precautions and clear the stretcher
- Discharge the paddles
  - When using defibrillation mode, the paddles discharge immediately

- When using synchronized cardioversion, there may be a delay until energy is timed with the patient's intrinsic electrical activity
- Monitor patient according to American Heart Association algorithms

Procedure 4
Instillation of Ear Drops and Ear Irrigation

INDICATIONS

- Delivery of medications (antibiotics, anticerumen agents, or steroid solutions)
- Irrigation of a foreign body or cerumen (for irrigation of ear, see Section III, Chapter 4 Eye, Ear, Nose, and Throat)

SUPPLIES

- Gloves
- Ear drops warmed to room temperature
  - Cold ear drops can cause increased pain
- Additional "holding" help as indicated

PROCEDURE

- Wash hands
- Apply gloves
- Maintain universal precautions
- Explain procedure in age-appropriate terminology
- Clean the outer ear if drainage or crusting is present
  - Do not attempt to clean the ear canal
    - Tympanic membrane rupture risk is high
- Position child with the ear to be instilled up
- For children <3 yr old, pull the pinna of the ear back and downward

- For children >3 yr old, pull the pinna of the ear back and upward
- Instill the ear drops as prescribed
- Keep child with ear up for at least several minutes
- Use cotton as needed
- Repeat procedure for other ear if drops are prescribed

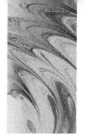

Procedure 5
Intraosseous Infusion*

INDICATIONS

- Vascular access in critically ill or injured child (age ≤6 yr) when unable to obtain peripheral IV within 90 sec or after three attempts, whichever occurs sooner

SUPPLIES

- Nonsterile gloves
- IO needle—may also use bone marrow needle or spinal needle
- Povidone-iodine solution
- Gauze 2 × 2s
- IV extension tubing
- Stopcock
- 5-mL or 10-mL syringe
- 60-mL syringe
- Tape
- IV tubing
- IV fluid to be administered
- Pressure infusion bag

PROCEDURE

- Localize insertion site (Fig. P5–1)
  - Preferred site is the flat, anteromedial surface of tibia, 1–3 cm below tibial tuberosity and just medial (may also use distal femur)
- Cleanse site

---

*Modified from Tipsord-Klinkhammer B, Andreoni C: Quick Reference for Emergency Nursing. Philadelphia, W.B. Saunders, 1998.

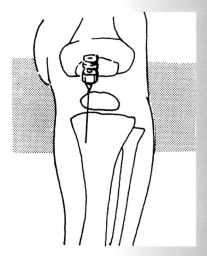

Figure P5–1. Insertion of intraosseous needle in the upper end of the tibia. (From McNeill M: Pediatric emergency procedures. *In* Singh N(ed): Manual of Pediatric Critical Care. Philadelphia, W.B. Saunders, 1997, p. 349.)

- Put on gloves; maintain universal precautions
- Insert intraosseous needle at a 90° angle, or slightly toward toes—to avoid growth plate; use a firm, twisting motion
  - Stabilize child's leg on a towel or folded blanket and hold with your nondominant hand, being careful not to have your hand behind insertion site
  - Insertion is often felt, and the needle will stand upright in the bone without support
- Withdraw stylet from needle
- Attach 5-mL or 10-mL syringe to needle and attempt to aspirate marrow
- Flush with 5–10 mL saline through IO needle
  - Assess resistance to flush and firmness of surrounding tissue
- Attach IV extension tubing to IO needle
- Place IV stopcock between extension tubing and IV administration tubing

- IV fluid boluses are administered by withdrawing IV solution into 60-mL syringe attached to the stopcock, closing stopcock to IV bag, and depressing plunger of syringe
- Attach pressure infusion bag to IV fluids
  - IO infusion by gravity is slow and inconsistent
- Stabilize IO needle by tape and gauze
- Continuously assess patency of IO needle and check for extravasation of fluid, medication

Procedure 6
Calculating Inotropic Medications Using the "Rule of Sixes"

INDICATIONS

- Accurate administration of inotropic medications to the critically ill or injured child (works best for children <20 kg)

SUPPLIES

- Medication ordered
- Buretrol
- IV tubing (for infusion pump) if using inline Buretrol
- 250-mL or 500-mL bag of 5% dextrose in water (D$_5$W)
- Calculator
- Tape or labels

PROCEDURE

- Determine child's weight in kilograms
- Review medication order for
  - Compatibility with current IV fluid infusing
  - Child's allergies
  - Appropriateness of dosage

Table P6–1. Calculation of Medications Using "Rule of Sixes"

	Dopamine Dobutamine Nitroprusside Nitroglycerine	Epinephrine Norepinephrine Isuprel Prostaglandin E$_1$	Lidocaine
Factor used to multiply the child's weight (kg)	6.0	0.6	60.0
Amount of medication to add to the Buretrol to a total of 100 mL fluid	6.0 × child's weight (kg)	0.6 × child's weight (kg)	60 × child's weight (kg)
Concentration of medication	1 mL/hr = 1 μg/kg/min	1 mL/hr = 0.1 μg/kg/min	1 mL/hr = 10 μg/kg/min

- Wash hands
- Insert Buretrol into IV bag of D_5W
- Attach IV tubing to Buretrol if using inline Buretrol
- Close roller clamp below Buretrol
- Open clamp above Buretrol and fill Buretrol with approximately 20 mL of D_5W, close clamp
  - Do *not* flush IV tubing below Buretrol with D_5W
- Calculate the amount of medication to add to the Buretrol according to Table P6–1
- Add medication to the Buretrol
- Fill Buretrol with D_5W to 100 mL, mix the solution gently
  - Do *not* add any more IV fluid or medication to the Buretrol until the Buretrol is completely empty
- Unclamp the IV tubing below the Buretrol and flush the IV tubing with the solution containing the inotropic medication
- Label the Buretrol with the medication added, the concentration, the date, the time, and your initials
- Label the infusion pump with the medication name and concentration
- Insert the IV tubing into the injection port (access site/stopcock) closest to the child
- Begin the infusion and titrate as per physician orders

IV Fluid Bolus Administration

INDICATIONS

- Rapid administration of IV fluids for volume replacement/fluid resuscitation

SUPPLIES

- Nonsterile gloves
- 60-mL syringe
- IV extension tubing
- Stopcock
- IV fluid (warmed if possible)
  - Crystalloid at 20 mL/kg initial bolus
  - Colloid (5% albumin or blood) at 10 mL/kg initial bolus
  - IV tubing

PROCEDURE

- Wash hands
- Put on gloves; maintain universal precautions
- Insert IV tubing into fluid to be administered
- Attach stopcock to end of IV tubing
- Attach extension tubing to stopcock
- Flush IV tubing, stopcock, and extension tubing
- Attach extension tubing to hub of IV catheter or IO needle
- Attach 60-mL syringe to third port of stopcock
- Turn stopcock off to child and open between IV bag and syringe
- Withdraw syringe plunger and draw up appropriate amount of fluid for the bolus from the IV bag

- Turn stopcock off to IV bag and open between syringe and child
- Administer IV fluid bolus by depressing plunger of syringe
- Turn stopcock off to syringe and open between child and IV bag
- Assess the effectiveness of fluid bolus
  - May repeat initial fluid bolus as ordered by physician
  - Return IV fluids to prescribed rate of infusion

IV Retrograde Medication Administration

INDICATIONS

- Administration of small amounts (<10 mL) of fluid containing medication over time
  - For example, antibiotics over 10–30 min

SUPPLIES

- Nonsterile gloves
- IV tubing with two injection ports (or access sites/stopcocks)
- Two 10-mL syringes
- 3-mL syringe
- Medication to be administered
- Antiseptic swabs
- Saline

PROCEDURE

- Review medication order for dosage and route
- Review allergies of child
- Review compatibility of medication with other medications, IV fluids infusing
- Determine the amount of fluid held in the IV tubing (check packaging if unsure)
  - Volume of reconstituted medication to be delivered should be no more than half of the total volume that the IV tubing holds
- Determine the infusion rate of the medication to be delivered

$$\frac{\text{Number of milliliters of reconstituted medication}}{\text{Number of minutes (time medication will infuse over)}} =$$

$$\frac{\text{Number of milliliters per hour (current IV infusion rate)}}{60 \text{ min (minutes in an hour)}}$$

- Wash hands
- Put on gloves; maintain universal precautions
- Clamp IV tubing between child and most proximal injection port (or access site/stopcock)
- Clamp IV tubing between most distal injection port and IV bag
- Insert 10-mL syringe into distal injection port
- Insert syringe with reconstituted medication into proximal injection port
- Slowly inject medication
  - The maintenance IV fluid is displaced out of the tubing and into the syringe in the distal injection port as the medication fills the tubing between each port
- Unclamp tubing in both places and remove syringes; medication will infuse by retrograde delivery
- Document medication administration

Procedure 9
Lumbar Puncture

INDICATIONS

- Rule out central nervous system infection
- Potential increased intracranial pressure (ICP) is ruled out prior to performance of lumbar puncture (LP)
- If any question of increased ICP due to bleeding, a computed tomography scan is obtained prior to LP

SUPPLIES

- LP tray or commercially available kit
- Adhesive bandage
- Antiseptic solution (Betadine)
- Sterile gloves
- Additional staff to assist with holding child, as indicated

PROCEDURE

- Wash hands
- Apply gloves
- Maintain universal precautions
- Proper positioning of the patient is crucial
  - Older child is placed near the edge of stretcher in lateral or sitting position; dangle legs over the side of the stretcher, bending over forward at the waist with the neck flexed; face the patient and hold in this position
  - Young infants may be held in sitting position; face the infant while holding an arm and leg in each of your hands

- Smaller child is placed in lateral position
  - Neck flexed and knees drawn upward (fetal position)
- Place one arm behind the patient's knees or thigh and the other behind the patient's neck
  - Avoid airway obstruction
  - Monitor heart rate and SpO_2 during procedure
- Be honest with older child about "bee sting" feeling during anesthetic injection
- Children <5 yr old will require a 22-gauge 1.5-inch needle
- After needle is removed, apply adhesive bandage
- Instruct older children to lie flat after the procedure
- Label cerebrospinal fluid (CSF) tubes as directed or as follows
  - Tube #1—culture and Gram's stain
  - Tube #2—protein and glucose
  - Tube #3—cell count
  - Tube #4—miscellaneous tests
- See Cerebrospinal Fluid Analysis Findings, Section I, Reference 7
- Observe child postprocedure for
  - Development of postprocedure headache (rare in small children and infants)
  - Leakage of CSF or blood from the puncture site

Procedure 10
Peripheral IV Insertion

INDICATIONS

- Administration of IV fluids or medications

SUPPLIES

- Nonsterile gloves
- Alcohol wipes
- Povidone-iodine solution
- Gauze 2 × 2s
- Tourniquet
- Appropriate-size armboard
- Tape
- Occlusive dressing
- IV fluid
- J-loop/T-connector
- IV extension tubing (check institutional policy)
- IV infusion pump—recommended for all pediatric IV infusions
- Saline flush solution prepared in 5-mL syringe
- Appropriate-size IV catheter
  - Butterfly needles may be used for scalp vein access
  - Over-the-needle catheters are preferred for peripheral lines; sizes range from 24–10 gauge
- Blood sampling equipment for specimen collection
  - Vacutainer tubes and transfer device for older child
  - 3-mL, 5-mL, or 10-mL syringes and 18- to 20-gauge needle for transfer of blood to tubes

PROCEDURE

- Explain procedure to child and parents
  - Consider the child's growth and developmental level
  - Be honest
- Explain parental role of support—*not* restraint
- Wash hands
- Put on gloves—maintain universal precautions
- Position child to avoid view of needles and procedure
- Determine best site for venipuncture—consider the following
  - Does child suck thumb?
  - Which is child's dominant hand?
  - Child's age
    - Infant: hand, antecubital fossa, foot, scalp
    - Young child: hand, antecubital fossa, foot
    - Older child: hand, antecubital fossa
- Consider applying armboard prior to venipuncture, if appropriate site
- Apply tourniquet, palpate vein, and choose puncture site
- Cleanse site per institutional policy
  - Generally, use povidone-iodine solution; allow to dry; use alcohol; allow to dry
- Insert needle with catheter with needle bevel up at 30–45° angle through skin just below vein
- Lower catheter and needle to 10–15° angle and advance toward the vein until a flashback is visualized
- Gently advance catheter while withdrawing needle
  - If catheter will not advance easily while flashback is present, remove needle and attach a T-connector/J-loop that has been flushed with saline to the catheter hub
  - Remove tourniquet and gently attempt to flush and "guide" catheter into vein with saline from syringe attached to end of connector

- Do *not* reinsert needle into catheter after it has been removed

BLOOD DRAW FOR SPECIMENS

- Only if saline has *not* been used to "guide" catheter into vein
- Infants and small children
  - Connect a 5-mL to 10-mL syringe to catheter hub, or to end of connector that is attached to catheter hub, and gently aspirate the amount of blood necessary for tests ordered
  - Immediately transfer blood from syringe to tubes using a 20-gauge or larger needle
- Older children
  - Connect Vacutainer transfer device with Vacutainer holder to hub of catheter and insert appropriate tubes for blood collection
  - Remove Vacutainer transfer device and attach connector to catheter hub
- Flush connector with saline and attach IV tubing (or IV extension tubing) to connector
- Administer IV fluids via IV infusion pump as ordered
- Stabilize IV catheter and apply occlusive dressing according to institutional policy
- Ensure proper immobilization of site by using armboard, gauze wrap, other devices that allow easy assessment of site for redness, swelling, dislodgment of catheter
- Reward child—consider growth and developmental level

Procedure 11

Use of Radiant Warmer Bed

INDICATIONS

- Provide warmth and maintain normothermia for ill or injured infants and neonates

SUPPLIES

- Radiant warmer with bed and temperature probe
- Infant blanket/sheet
- Manufacturer's instructions

PROCEDURE

- Radiant warmer bed should always be plugged in and turned on to prewarm setting while not in use
- Explain procedure/use of radiant warmer bed to parents
- Wash hands
- Prewarm the radiant warmer bed and blanket
  - Turn control to manual setting
  - Set power level to 100%
- Prepare for placement of infant in warmer bed
  - Turn control to servo—this will automatically adjust the heat delivered, maintaining a constant skin temperature
    - Do not place infant in warmer bed with controls on manual—burns may occur
  - Set control temperature (window display of numbers) on warmer control panel to 37°C (98.6°F)

- Cover bed mattress with infant blanket or sheet
- Place undressed infant on bed
  - Do not cover infant with clothing or linens
- Insert temperature probe into warmer and place flat metal side of probe next to infant's skin at right upper quadrant (over area of infant's liver)
  - Use reflective thermal probe cover to adhere probe to infant's skin
- Observe patient temperature (window display of infant's skin temperature) on warmer control panel
  - Alarm will be activated if skin temperature varies 1°C more or less than set control temperature
- Obtain axillary temperature of infant when placed in bed and repeat in 15 min
- Obtain axillary temperature every 2 hr and document patient temperature and control temperature from control panel of radiant warmer

Procedure 12

Specimen Collection for Respiratory Syncytial Virus

INDICATIONS

- To collect specimen via nasal washing to identify the presence of respiratory syncytial virus (RSV)

SUPPLIES

- Butterfly needle
- Scissors
- Nonsterile gloves
- Viral transport medium
- 3- to 5-mL syringe
- 1–4 mL sterile saline

PROCEDURE

- Explain procedure to child and parents
- Explain parental role of support—*not* restraint
- Wash hands
- Put on gloves; maintain universal precautions
- Draw up 1–4 mL sterile saline into syringe through butterfly needle
- Using scissors, cut needle from butterfly device
- Position child upright—on stretcher or on parent's lap
- Insert plastic tubing gently through child's nare into nasopharynx; instill saline solution (~2 mL)

- Immediately withdraw plunger of syringe, aspirating nasal secretions as the tubing is withdrawn from the child's nare
- Transfer nasal washing specimen to appropriate viral transport medium
- Offer the child tissue for nose
- Reward child for cooperation—consider age and developmental level

Procedure 13
Spinal Immobilization

INDICATIONS

- To correctly immobilize the spine in the injured child when the mechanism of injury and/or child's condition indicates the risk of a spinal injury

SUPPLIES

- Nonsterile gloves
- Long backboard with straps
  - Pediatric molded backboards are commercially available
- Towel rolls/blanket roll
- Rigid cervical collar
- Towel or infant blanket
- Tape

PROCEDURE

- Obtain assistance
- Put on gloves; maintain universal precautions
- Manually immobilize the child as assistants are preparing supplies
  - Stand behind the head of the stretcher
  - Place one hand on each side of child's head
  - Thumb stabilizes mandible, and fingers spread across the occiput
  - Stabilize and immobilize—do *not* apply traction
  - Maintain head in a neutral, inline position
  - Avoid hyperflexion or hyperextension
  - Do not remove manual immobilization (with

　　　　your hands) until child is definitively immobi-
　　　　lized
- Perform a brief neurologic examination
    - AVPU assessment (see Section III, Chapter
      10 Neurologic)
    - Motor strength of extremities—consider age
      and developmental level
- Assistant—apply rigid cervical collar *only* if appropriate-size collar is available
    - Child's chin should fit into chin groove of col-
      lar
    - Collar should not cover child's ears
    - Do *not* hyperextend or hyperflex the child's
      neck to fit into collar
    - If appropriate-size collar is not available, use
      a rolled towel or sheet to fashion a soft collar
        - A peri pad or large abdominal dressing
          may be used as a collar for infants
- With assistants, place child onto long backboard
    - Continue to maintain manual immobilization
    - The person immobilizing the head and neck
      is the leader and directs the assistants
    - Backboard is placed next to child
        - When a flat board is used, a folded towel
          or infant blanket is placed at the level of
          the infant's shoulders to prevent flexion of
          neck due to the large occiput of infants
    - Log-roll the child as one unit, sliding the
      backboard under the child as he or she is
      turned
- Secure the child to the backboard by straps
    - Continue manual immobilization
    - Pad the large backboard laterally (if using
      adult-size board) with linen to prevent small
      child from moving about despite the straps
- Secure the head by using towel rolls or a blan-
  ket roll on each side of the child's head
    - Do *not* use sandbags or IV fluid bags
- Tape across child's forehead, including the
  towel rolls and securing the tape to the board

- Do not tape across the chin or use gauze under tape against skin
- Discontinue manual immobilization now that child is definitively immobilized
- Repeat a brief neurologic examination
  - AVPU assessment
  - Motor strength of extremities—consider age and development of child
- Reward child for cooperation—consider age and developmental level

Procedure 14
Application of Splints

INDICATIONS

- Stabilization of fracture
- Prevents further damage to nerves and blood vessels
- Decreases pain

SUPPLIES

- There are various types of splints used for specific types of fractures or severe sprains
  - Clavicle strap
  - Soft: pillow, sling
  - Rigid: posterior plaster, polymer, or fiberglass mold; air splint; metal; hard plastic
  - Traction
    - Thomas
    - Hare
    - Bucks
- If closed reduction of a forearm/wrist is necessary, supplies for a Bier block include
  - IV access (small-gauge butterfly needle may be adequate and less painful)
  - Padding for upper arm (cast padding works well)
  - Latex wrap (check for latex sensitivity; sometimes used to wrap from distal to proximal arm to push blood upward)
  - Blood pressure cuff (to be inflated to approximately 30–50 mm Hg above child's systolic blood pressure)
  - Preservative-free lidocaine diluted to 0.125%

- Supplies for posterior mold application
  - Water
  - Cast padding (if indicated)
  - Elastic bandage(s)
  - Splinting material (many commercial brands available)
  - Scissors

PROCEDURE FOR POSTERIOR MOLDED SPLINT APPLICATION

- Wash hands
- Put on gloves
- Measure the splint material as indicated (Figs. P14–1 to P14–5)
- Pad the arm with cast padding (if indicated—some commercial products no longer require padding)
- Wet the splint material (dip in water or use a water bottle) and remove excess water
- Apply the splint as required by type of fracture
- Wrap elastic bandage over the splint to secure the position
  - Make sure elastic wrap is not too tight
- Check circulation distal to fracture site
- Allow splint to become firm
  - Splint may become warm during the firming stage
- Apply ice bags over fracture site for first 24–48 hr after injury

1. Measure from 1 inch above
   the palmar crease to 2 inches
   from the antecubital. Prepare
   splint as directed.

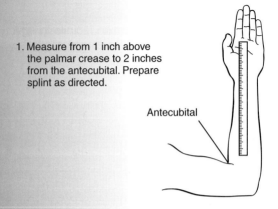

Antecubital

2. Fold one edge of the splint
   over 1 inch. Place fold at the
   angle of the palmar crease.
   (Follow the life line.)

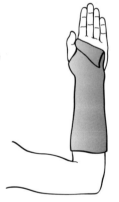

Figure P14–1. Volar splint. (From Ortho-Glass® Splinting
Manual. Charlotte, NC, Smith & Nephew, 1995.)

3. Wrap with elastic bandage to secure the splint. Mold and position as prescribed by physician.

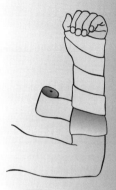

Figure P14–1 *Continued.*

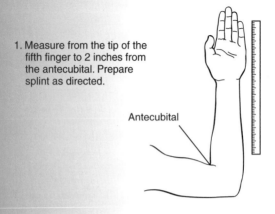

1. Measure from the tip of the fifth finger to 2 inches from the antecubital. Prepare splint as directed.

Antecubital

2. Place padding between the fourth and fifth fingers.

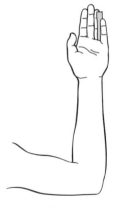

Figure P14–2. Boxer splint. (From Ortho-Glass® Splinting Manual. Charlotte, NC, Smith & Nephew, 1995.)

3. Apply the splint to the ulnar side of the hand, creating a gutter.

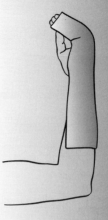

4. Wrap with elastic bandage to secure the splint. Mold and position as prescribed by physician.

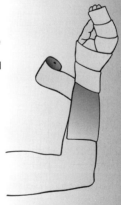

Figure P14–2 *Continued.*

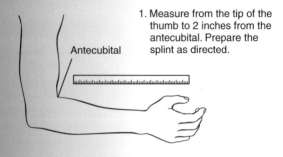

1. Measure from the tip of the thumb to 2 inches from the antecubital. Prepare the splint as directed.

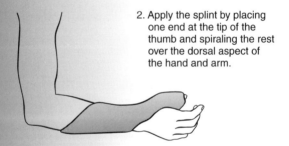

2. Apply the splint by placing one end at the tip of the thumb and spiraling the rest over the dorsal aspect of the hand and arm.

Figure P14–3. Thumb spica splint. (From Ortho-Glass® Splinting Manual. Charlotte, NC, Smith & Nephew, 1995.)

3. Wrap by starting at the wrist and making two figure-eight wraps around the thumb.

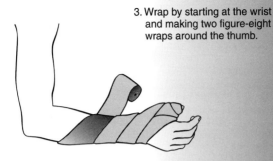

4. Mold and position as prescribed by physician.

Figure P14–3 *Continued.*

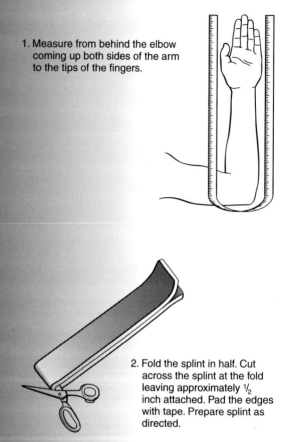

1. Measure from behind the elbow coming up both sides of the arm to the tips of the fingers.

2. Fold the splint in half. Cut across the splint at the fold leaving approximately ½ inch attached. Pad the edges with tape. Prepare splint as directed.

Figure P14–4. Reverse sugar-tong splint. (From Ortho-Glass® Splinting Manual. Charlotte, NC, Smith & Nephew, 1995.)

3. Place the splint on the patient's arm by sliding the cut section over the fingers with the attached section in the web space between the thumb and forefinger.

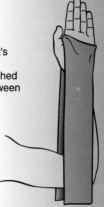

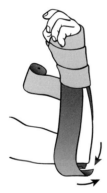

4. Wrap with elastic bandage to secure the splint. At the elbow, fold one side of the excess material behind the elbow and overlap with the other side. Lock in place with a series of figure-eight wraps.

Figure P14–4 *Continued.*

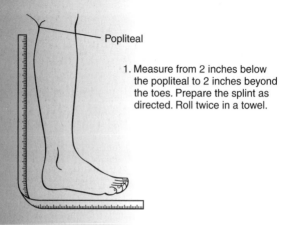

Popliteal

1. Measure from 2 inches below the popliteal to 2 inches beyond the toes. Prepare the splint as directed. Roll twice in a towel.

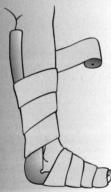

2. Fold the splint under 1 inch at the toes to make a reinforcing toe plate. Place the splint under the foot, extending slightly beyond the toes and wrap as follows: Start at the toes, work up the foot, skip the ankle, and wrap behind the achilles.

Figure P14–5. Posterior ankle splint. (From Ortho-Glass® Splinting Manual. Charlotte, NC, Smith & Nephew, 1995.)

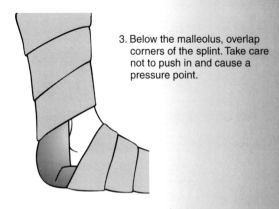

3. Below the malleolus, overlap corners of the splint. Take care not to push in and cause a pressure point.

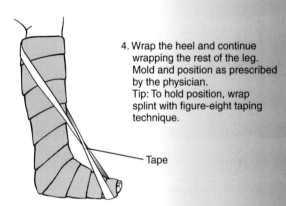

4. Wrap the heel and continue wrapping the rest of the leg. Mold and position as prescribed by the physician.
Tip: To hold position, wrap splint with figure-eight taping technique.

— Tape

Figure P14–5 *Continued.*

Procedure 15
Central Venous Access Device

INDICATIONS

- Intermittent infusions or long-term IV access for the chronically ill child
- Infusions for a required time frame that exceeds time periods for peripheral IV catheters
- Includes tunneled, nontunneled, implanted medication ports, and peripherally inserted central catheters
- Used for
  - IV therapy
  - Chemotherapy
  - Medication
  - Blood products
  - Blood sampling
  - Parenteral nutrition

SUPPLIES

- Use only noncore needles with an implanted venous access device (VAD)
  - Right-angle noncoring needle is very common
  - 19-gauge for blood infusion or withdrawal
  - 20-gauge for most other infusions
- Syringes (5-mL or larger)
- Sterile normal saline for injection (preservative-free for infants <12 mo old)
- Heparin solution for injection (preservative-free for infants <12 mo old)
- Sterile gloves and mask
- Medications, blood, or nutritional product for injection

- Laboratory tubes if blood sampling is ordered

PROCEDURE

- Wash hands
- Apply gloves and mask
- Maintain a sterile field around the device
- Prepare the site prior to access—refer to institutional policy
- For implanted devices/medication ports
  - Palpate the area to locate the implanted VAD
  - Insert the needle at the center of the device perpendicular to the port if top access device, and parallel if side-entry access device; push through the skin and port until the needle touches bottom of the VAD reservoir
  - Aspirate for blood return
  - If unable to aspirate blood or flush the VAD, trouble shoot for
    - Kinked tubing
    - Closed clamp
    - Kinked catheter
- For all VADs, after successful infusion, flush the central line
  - Always aspirate and flush with a 5-mL or larger syringe to prevent catheter damage from excessive pressure created by a smaller syringe
  - Flush with 2 mL sterile saline
  - Follow with heparin flush
    - For infants <12 mo, flush with 1 mL heparin solution (100 units/mL)
    - For children >12 mo or >5 kg, flush with 2 mL of heparin solution (100 units/mL)
- Monitor for
  - Site infection
  - Skin breakdown
  - Extravasation of injected fluid
  - Phlebitis

Selected Bibliography

Ashwill JW, Droske SC: Nursing Care of Children: Principles and Practice. Philadelphia, W.B. Saunders, 1997.

Barkin R, Rosen P: Emergency Pediatrics: A Guide to Ambulatory Care, 4th ed. St. Louis, Mosby–Year Book, 1994.

French J: Pediatric Emergency Skills. St. Louis, Mosby–Year Book, 1995.

Haley K, Baker P (eds): Instructor Manual: Emergency Nursing Pediatric Course. Chicago, Emergency Nurses Association, 1993.

Singh N: Manual of Pediatric Critical Care. Philadelphia, W.B. Saunders, 1997.

Soud TE, Rogers JS: Manual of Pediatric Emergency Nursing. Philadelphia, Mosby–Year Book, 1998.

Tipsord-Klinkhammer B, Andreoni C: Quick Reference for Emergency Nursing. Philadelphia, W.B. Saunders, 1998.

Index

Note: Page numbers in *italics* refer to illustrations; page numbers followed by t refer to tables.

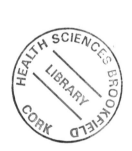

Pediatric Modification of Glasgow Coma Scale (GCS) by Age of Patient*

Glasgow Coma Score

Pediatric Modification

Eye opening

≥1 year

4 Spontaneously
3 To verbal command
2 To pain
1 No response

0–1 yr

4 Spontaneously
3 To shout
2 To pain
1 No response

Best motor response

≥1 year

6 Obeys
5 Localizes pain
4 Flexion withdrawal
3 Flexion abnormal (decorticate posturing)

2 Extension (decerebrate posturing)

1 No response

0–1 yr

6 Normal spontaneous movements
5 Localizes pain
4 Flexion withdrawal
3 Flexion abnormal (decorticate posturing)
2 Extension (decerebrate posturing)
1 No response